# THE CHOLESTEROL DELUSION

## By Ernest N. Curtis, MD

First published by Dog Ear Publishing
4010 W. 86th Street, Ste H
Indianapolis, IN 46268
www.dogearpublishing.net

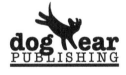

ISBN: 978-160844-748-0

This book is printed on acid-free paper.

Printed in the United States of America

Delusion: A false belief or wrong judgment held with conviction despite incontrovertible evidence to the contrary.

Stedman's Medical Dictionary

# TABLE OF CONTENTS

# GLOSSARY

AHA      American Heart Association

AS      <u>Atherosclerosis</u>: A degenerative disease involving the large and medium sized arteries characterized by the development of plaques within the arterial wall.

CAD      <u>Coronary artery disease</u>: Atherosclerosis involving the coronary arteries.

CHD      <u>Coronary heart disease</u>: Disorders of the heart caused by complications of AS in the coronary arteries. Includes heart attack (MI) and chest pains known as angina pectoris.

<u>Cholesterol Theory</u>: A subset of the Risk Factor Theory. The concept that the cholesterol level in the blood is the chief causative factor in AS.

<u>Diet-Heart Theory</u>: The idea that saturated fats and cholesterol in the diet cause AS of the coronary arteries and subsequent coronary heart disease.

<u>Lipid</u>: A descriptive term for substances which are insoluble in water and soluble in fat solvents such as alcohol, ether, or chloroform. Includes true fats, lipoids, and sterols.

MI      <u>Myocardial Infarction</u>: Technical term for heart attack. Complete blockage of a branch of the coronary arteries causes death of the muscle cells in that part of the heart served by that artery.

NFMI      <u>Nonfatal Myocardial Infarction</u>: A heart attack from which the victim survives.

NIH         <u>National Institutes of Health</u>: Official agency of the federal government whose function is to fund and conduct research related to health and disease.

NLHBI       <u>National Heart, Lung, and Blood Institute</u>: A major branch of the NIH that controls government funding of cardiovascular research.

            <u>Plaque</u>: A lesion within the arterial wall characterized by a proliferation of cells that form a fibrous cap.

            <u>Risk Factors</u>: Characteristics or conditions that show a positive correlation with a disease. Often mistakenly thought of as causes of the disease.

            <u>Thrombosis</u>: Development of blood clots.

# FOREWORD

This book grew out of a talk I gave at some medical education seminars almost thirty years ago. Having developed an interest in cardiology during my second or third year in medical school, I was always interested in the latest theories on coronary artery disease and heart attacks. During this time, the "risk factor" concept was accepted as the key to prevention and treatment of coronary heart disease. This theory postulated a number of factors that would predispose an individual to develop coronary artery disease and therefore be at risk for heart attack.

Clearly, some of the risk was genetic, as the occurrence of premature heart attacks was known to run in families. But other causes were said to be due to external influences that individuals could control by modification of their behavior. Most prominent among these were cigarette smoking and a diet too high in saturated fats and cholesterol. This theory seemed reasonable and, as far as I knew, was generally accepted; however, my doubts began to arise after I entered my postgraduate training. I was fortunate to take my medical residency and cardiology fellowship in the mid-1970s at a large community hospital with an active cardiology department. Thus, I was able to see and learn from hundreds of patients who suffered from coronary heart disease.

There was only one problem. Most of the patients I was seeing did not fit the "risk factor" profile I had been taught. In fact, more than a few patients plaintively asked, "How can I be having a heart attack?" or said, "I don't smoke or eat red meat," or, "I exercise daily," etc.

I would answer that the risk factors were based on probabilities and, naturally, there would be some exceptions. But I was seeing far too many exceptions for my own peace of mind and felt the need to understand more. Therefore, I started haunting the medical library during my free time. I was surprised to discover that a few articles here and there disagreed vehemently with the prevalent theories—especially that about the relationship of coronary heart disease to diet. These dissident arguments raised some very good questions and made me want to explore the origins of the prevailing theories to see if the evidence was convincing.

I submitted an application for a Medline search on the topics of diet, cholesterol, and coronary heart disease. This generated a list of more than 500 medical journal articles and reviews. Most of these were available in our own medical library, and the rest I obtained through an interlibrary copy service. I found that examination of the references cited by these articles led back to the original studies upon which the Cholesterol Theory was based. I was surprised at how weak and sometimes virtually nonexistent the evidence was for this theory.. But no matter how long I searched, the articles and reviews all ultimately referred back to the same "evidence" as the foundation for the theory.

At that time, the country was in the grip of a cholesterol mania, so I decided to put together a presentation detailing the arguments and evidence against the cholesterol theory. This developed into a two-hour talk that I delivered on a few occasions to groups of medical and family practice residents at our hospital. I also spoke at a few local service clubs and community organizations as part of our hospital's speaker program. The response was somewhat underwhelming, but I attributed that to my own deficiencies as a speaker. I toyed with the idea of putting the information I had gathered into a book, but because I was just starting my medical practice, there was really no time to do so.

As the years went by, I continually counseled my patients to eat what they liked, ignore their cholesterol levels, and avoid cholesterol-lowering drugs like the plague. Most listened politely but probably disregarded what I was saying because "everybody knew" that diet and cholesterol were important. People heard it every day and read it on all the labels of the foods they bought. Still, I really didn't fret a great deal because I figured that all I could do was provide the information. People would do with it what they wished.

Ironically, what changed my attitude was watching the evolution of the campaign against cigarette smoking. When it became evident that education on the health risks of smoking wouldn't stamp it out completely, the anti-smoking forces turned to the coercive arm of the government. They started with dramatic warning labels on cigarette packs and then got a legislative ban on cigarette advertising. Finally, through the use of "junk science," they were able to convince enough of the right people that secondhand smoke was an actual health hazard to nonsmokers. This opened the floodgates for laws and regulations to be passed and huge "sin" taxes to be imposed. Initially, anti-smoking activists lobbied only for a ban on smoking in small enclosed places like airplanes; however, this was incrementally extended to include restaurants and other "public" places. Today we see legislatures and local city councils passing laws banning smoking outdoors and in people's private homes!

We have, in a short time, seen the act of smoking progress from an annoying habit to a sin and, finally, to a vicious health hazard that supposedly disables and kills innocent people. Incredibly, we now have courts of law awarding people huge monetary judgments for the medical consequences of something they freely chose to do despite the ubiquitous publicity and exhortations against it.

One might ask what all this has to do with the diet-heart business. Well, the food fascists are following the path blazed by the anti-smoking forces. The "junk science" incriminating high-cholesterol and high-fat foods has been in place for years. Extensive labeling of food products has already been accomplished. There have been proposals to ban certain foods in public schools and to put a prohibitive tax on "unhealthy" food for the general public. Keep in mind how far the incremental changes in smoking regulation have taken us. I predict that class action lawsuits against food producers and servers are not far off. These noxious possibilities looming on the horizon motivated me to write this book.

My goal is to persuade you, the reader, that your cholesterol level and the foods you eat have nothing to do with the development of atherosclerosis and coronary heart disease. To this end, I have tried to avoid unnecessary technical jargon wherever possible. I provide a glossary of terms and abbreviations that will be frequently used to aid your understanding of the topics discussed in this book. Because this book is meant to be a survey of the topic for the general public, I have avoided the temptation to overload the reader with scientific references—especially on points that are scientifically settled. For example, most people are surprised to learn that diet has virtually no effect on blood cholesterol levels and that there is really no debate about this among knowledgeable scientists. Rather than list several of the hundreds of references on this point, I have listed a number of books in the bibliography at the end of this book. There the reader can find ample documentation on points he or she feels are inadequately covered in this book..

People sometimes ask me, "Why should I believe you when your statements and conclusions go against everything we've been told for years?" My response is the same as I give to you, the reader: Don't take my word for it. But don't take anyone else's, either, unless they've done the research and have no vested interest in the current dogma. I would urge everyone to examine the evidence cited by the proponents of the Diet-Heart and Cholesterol Theories that are referenced in the text of this book. Look at the key articles that claim to prove the theory in question and see if the evidence stands up to critical examination.* I have written a brief guide on how to read and interpret medical journal articles in the appendices to help those who want to delve deeper but aren't familiar with scientific literature.

I realize that many of you have only a superficial or passing interest in this subject and therefore won't want to pursue it in any depth. But I would strongly advise anyone who is taking or has been advised to take drugs to lower their cholesterol to expend the time and effort to verify what is presented here. Your life may literally depend on it.

*Appendices II and III contain the medical journal articles reporting on the two clinical trials most often cited as definitively proving the cholesterol theory.

# CHAPTER ONE

## THE THEORY DEFINED

*"It ain't what you don't know that can hurt you; it's what you do know that ain't true."*

Artemus Ward

What do the following statements have in common?

1) Heart attack is the leading cause of death in the US today.

2) Heart attacks are caused by a buildup of cholesterol plaques inside the coronary arteries.

3) Cholesterol plaques are caused by an elevated level of cholesterol in the blood.

4) A high-fat, high-cholesterol diet will raise the blood cholesterol level and thus put a person at risk for coronary artery disease, eventually leading to heart attack and, likely, premature death.

5) Lowering the cholesterol level with diet and/or drugs will decrease the risk of developing coronary artery disease, prevent heart attacks, and save countless lives

What these statements have in common is:1) They are commonly accepted as true and, 2) They are entirely wrong; that is, they are not supported by a shred of scientifically credible evidence

Taken together, these ideas comprise what is commonly known as the Lipid Hypothesis, or the Cholesterol Theory, of atherosclerosis and heart disease. The linkage to dietary fat and cholesterol is known as the Diet-Heart Theory. This theory, which had its origins in the 19th century, began to be seriously pushed in the 1950s and 1960s by a group of proponents who were dedicated to the idea that diet is the cause of atherosclerosis and coronary heart disease These people ultimately came into control of the American Heart Association(AHA) and the National Heart Lung and Blood Institute (NHLBI), the two institutions responsible for almost all funding of research in heart disease. The NHLBI is a major division of the National Institutes of Health (NIH) and therefore determines who gets funded with taxpayer dollars. The AHA is the primary fundraising organization for private donations. These two groups also provide the bulk of the information on heart disease and research that gets conveyed to the public through the media.

By the 1970s and 1980s, the Cholesterol Theory had achieved the status of accepted dogma both within the medical profession and with the general public. The critics of the theory have maintained that it is based on faulty premises, unreliable statistical data, and unscientific analysis. Unfortunately such a huge vested interest has grown around this theory that the critics are rarely heard.

The purpose of this book is to show that the proponents of the Cholesterol Theory are wrong and the critics correct. Let me, at the outset, state my position as clearly and unequivocally as possible. The Cholesterol Theory and the Diet-Heart Theory are scientifically bankrupt. Moreover, the continued presentation of these unproven theories as established fact in both the popular press and medical journals causes  harm by diverting attention from the true causes and wasting billions of dollars on useless research. The Cholesterol Theory is a near-perfect medical analog of the Emperor's New Clothes: When examined closely, there is nothing there. Proof of a causal link between cholesterol and coronary heart disease (CHD) is completely lacking. Proof of the efficacy of lowering cholesterol at reducing the incidence of CHD and thus saving lives is equally lacking. Objective review of the evidence can lead only to the conclusion that the Cholesterol Theory and all of its ancillary baggage such as low-fat diets and cholesterol-lowering drugs should be thrown into the ashcan of medical history and then jumped on with both feet.

I will not attempt to prove that the Cholesterol and Diet-Heart Theories are false. Those of you who are familiar with the formal study of logic know that it is not logically possible to prove a negative construct but rather, the burden of proof always lies with the one who makes a positive assertion. I will therefore trace the development of the Cholesterol Theory from its origin and apply scientific reasoning and analysis to the evidence given by the proponents to see if it holds up under critical scrutiny. This is best done by taking the studies cited most often by the proponents as proving the Cholesterol Theory and examining them in some detail.

But first, it is necessary to present the basics of coronary artery disease and heart attacks so it is clear what the subsequent discussion is all about.

## CHAPTER TWO

# CARDIOLOGY 101:
# THE HEART AND HEART ATTACKS

The heart is a muscular pump whose proper functioning is essential to the body's circulatory system and, thus, to life itself. It is, in many ways, the most remarkable organ in the human body. To gain a proper appreciation for the job the heart does, try contracting (flexing) your biceps muscle about sixty times per minute and see how long you can sustain this activity. The muscle that forms the walls of the heart contracts an average of 60 to 100 times per minute every minute of the day and night. Moreover, it can continue this for up to 100 or more years without ever stopping. Unlike the other muscles of the body, the heart can never take a rest. Should it stop, death of the individual would ensue in a few short moments.

In order to perform this function, the heart needs a constant supply of oxygen, energy, and nutrients, which are all carried in the bloodstream. The chief function of the heart is to pump the blood throughout the body to all the muscles and organs, including the heart itself. The conduits for this blood supply consist of a system of tubular blood vessels of two different types known as arteries and veins.

The arteries are relatively thick-walled tubes through which the heart pumps oxygenated blood to all the muscles and vital organs. The veins are thin-walled vessels that return the oxygen-depleted blood back to the heart and lungs under low pressure.

The walls of the arteries are thick because they must transmit and contain the strong pumping force of the heart. The pressure in the arteries may range from 90 to 200 mmHg(Millimeters of mercury;this is the number measured by a blood pressure cuff placed on the arm), while that in the veins is usually around 2 to 5 mmHg.

Much of the thickness and strength of the arterial wall are provided by a middle layer of smooth muscle that is oriented circumferentially. This means that the smooth muscle encircles the perimeter of the arterial tube much like a belt encircles one's waist or the equator encircles the earth. With this orientation contraction of the muscle will narrow the diameter of the artery and, therefore, somewhat restrict the flow of blood through it. Relaxation of the muscle allows the artery to enlarge or dilate thereby facilitating a greater flow of blood. This is similar to the way a camera's diaphragm will control the size of the aperture to allow more or less light to enter as needed. The pupil of the eye will constrict or dilate in the same fashion. This is important because it allows the body to shunt arterial blood flow to areas where it is most needed. For example, following a meal, the arteries to the skin will constrict and those to the intestines will dilate, thus diverting arterial blood away from the skin, where it is not needed, and toward the intestines, which are now working hard to digest and absorb the food.

In similar fashion, heavy physical exercise will constrict the arteries to the intestines and other organs, where blood flow is less necessary, and dilate those to the working muscles. Thus, the arterial blood flow can be shifted and redirected so that blood flow is greatly increased in response to increased demand in certain areas and reduced where the demand is low.

The blood that brings oxygen and nutrients to the heart flows through the coronary arteries. If the flow of blood to a portion of the heart is interrupted, that portion of the heart will begin to die from lack of oxygen. This death of a portion of the heart muscle is known as myocardial infarction (MI), what is commonly known as a heart attack. A few minutes' interruption in the blood flow is usually enough to start this process.

There are two main coronary arteries (called left and right) and several branches of these, which go to different parts of the heart. Anything that cuts off the flow of blood in either of the main arteries or the sub-branches can cause a heart attack in that portion of the heart served by that particular branch. The damaged area will heal by forming scar tissue, similar to that seen in other wounds. The part of the heart muscle that has become scar tissue can no longer participate in the pumping of the heart. If the area of damage is small, overall heart function will not be greatly affected. If the area of damage is large, however, the heart will not be able to pump as efficiently as before and the victim will experience a reduction in his ability to perform physical activities. The reduction may be moderate or severe, depending on the extent of the damage.

The cutting off of blood flow in a coronary artery is caused by the development of a blood clot in a portion of the artery that has been previously narrowed by atherosclerosis (AS). Atherosclerosis may also be called arteriosclerosis or "hardening of the arteries." Although there are some differences in the precise definitions of these terms, for our purposes, we can treat them as equivalent. AS is a degenerative disease process that affects primarily the large- and medium-sized arteries. (A degenerative disease is one that occurs mainly through wear and tear over time as we grow older.)

Atherosclerosis is ubiquitous. It is found in all animal species and in humans of all ages. During the Korean War in the early 1950s, a team of army doctors set out to examine wound ballistics in soldiers killed in action. They performed more than 2000 autopsies and were shocked to find that practically all soldiers showed evidence of AS in varying degrees of severity. Almost half of the soldiers autopsied had coronary arterial lesions graded as moderately severe or worse. These men not only were young (average age 22 years) but also had undergone a rigorous physical training prior to their deployment in the field.

The International Atherosclerosis Project examined more than 25,000 arterial specimens submitted by pathologists from all over the world and concluded that, although there were differences in severity, no individual or population group was free of the disease. Investigators have found evidence of early AS in almost all infants and young children. They have even chronicled some of the earliest changes in fetuses. Atherosclerosis is also widely spread throughout the animal kingdom. Almost no species is spared. This includes both carnivores and herbivores. Long-lived species such as chimpanzees, gorillas, and parrots have shown severe AS despite their almost exclusively vegetarian diet.

Atherosclerosis is characterized by the development of multiple fibrous plaques within the inner walls of the arteries. These plaques develop within the arterial wall, between the thin inner coating called the endothelium and the thicker muscular layer in the middle portion of the wall. This is in direct contrast to the common conception of fats and cholesterol deposited directly on the inner lining of the artery much like sludge in a pipe. This point requires special emphasis: **There is nothing deposited on or sticking to the inside of the arterial wall**. Something stimulates smooth muscle cells from the middle layer of the arterial wall to migrate inward and proliferate into successive sheets of cells. These smooth muscle cells form a fibrous plaque that will rigidify that portion of the previously pliable arterial wall. As the plaque enlarges, it will push into the path of the blood flow and progressively narrow the internal diameter of the artery.[1]  Generally, there is no noticeable reduction in blood flow until the arterial diameter is at least 70% reduced meaning the blood must now squeeze through an area only ¼ to 1/3 the diameter of a normal artery. Some plaques are prone to develop cracks and fissures and may even rupture. Any of these complications may trigger blood clotting, which can then completely block the artery and cause a heart attack.

The disruption of the plaque, which causes the blood clot and thus the heart attack is a rather sudden and abrupt event.[2]  Cracking or rupture of the surface of the plaque will expose the underlying layer of collagen to the circulating blood. This will usually initiate the blood clotting process through the activation of tiny particles in the blood called platelets. Platelets are manufactured in the bone marrow and act as the first responders to any injury. Normally, they circulate as discrete particles,but chemicals released from a site of injury  will  cause the platelets to clump together and form an initial plug at the site of injury. Then certain proteins in the blood (called clotting factors) will gradually form a mature clot around the plug formed by the clumped platelets.

Although most people with AS have multiple plaques, only one plaque at a time will trigger this sudden event. Even more interesting is the fact that in most heart attacks, it isn't the largest or most significantly obstructive plaque that cracks or ruptures and starts the process. Recent studies in which angiograms have been done before and after heart attack have shown that relatively minor plaques are often the initiators.[3] In fact, only 1/3 of heart attacks occur in the site deemed most likely prior to the event (the largest or most obstructive plaques). This is important, because the cause of the underlying AS may have nothing to do with the cause of the plaque disruption that leads to the heart attack. The proponents of the Cholesterol Theory maintain that cholesterol is the main causative factor in the development of AS. They have no clue as to what triggers the plaque changes that lead directly to heart attack (and, in fairness, neither does anyone else).

The crucial point here is that we are dealing with two separate phenomena—the gradual development of AS over time and the relatively sudden disruption of a previously stable plaque that triggers the heart attack. Although the process of AS certainly sets the stage for the heart attack, the proximate cause of the heart attack may be completely unrelated. These important differences must be kept in mind when we examine the various studies cited as supporting the Cholesterol Theory. These studies invariably use "end points" or outcomes that include deaths from coronary heart disease (CHD deaths) and nonfatal myocardial infarctions (NFMI). Even if cholesterol were a causative factor in AS (which it isn't), that has nothing to do with whatever may cause the acute changes in plaque stability that lead to heart attack.

Because the subject of "cardiac death" or "sudden death" will play a large role in the studies we will examine, it is appropriate here to examine a few points relevant to that subject. Death from a heart attack is almost never due to the direct damage to the muscle cells. Although a small percentage of people with heart attack may die from rupture of the damaged muscle, most die because of a heart rhythm disturbance. The damaged muscle brings about an instability in the heart's electrical system, which results in a rhythm disturbance (arrhythmia) known as ventricular fibrillation. The disordered electrical impulses in ventricular fibrillation cause the heart to merely "twitch" rather than contract in the normal and regular rhythm that provides adequate blood flow.. Without the central pumping function of the heart, there is complete cessation of blood flow to the entire body and death within a very short time.

These deaths usually occur outside the hospital and are often unwitnessed. The problem is that there are a number of other causes of sudden death that have nothing to do with the heart or coronary artery disease. These may range from drug-induced deaths to ruptured cerebral aneurysm. A substantial percentage of sudden deaths show no discernible cause despite a detailed autopsy examination. Unfortunately, there is a tendency to label almost all sudden unexpected deaths as heart attacks; this tendency will, of course, distort the statistics. Because almost all the studies we will examine use "death from coronary heart disease" as one of their chief end points, it is important to determine how the authors of any given study decide which deaths fit that category.

With this background information on AS and CHD, let's now turn to Cholesterol Theory to explore its origins and evolution and examine the evidence offered by its proponents.

# CHAPTER THREE

# WHAT IS THIS THING CALLED CHOLESTEROL?

*"Ignorance is preferable to error, and he is less remote from the truth who believes nothing than he who believes what is wrong."*

Thomas Jefferson

Cholesterol is one of the most vital and important biochemical compounds in nature. It is a major component of every cell in the body. All cells are enclosed by a membrane that keeps the contents of the cell intact and regulates everything that enters or leaves the cell. One can think of the cell membrane as the protective coat of the cell, regulating the inflow of fluids and nutrients and keeping out unwanted invaders. All cell membranes are composed of cholesterol and cholesterol-derived compounds. Brain and nerve tissue contain the highest proportion of cholesterol in the body.

Cholesterol is the basic building block for the formation of bile acids which are essential for the proper digestion and absorption of many foods. Without cholesterol and the bile acids derived from it, we couldn't absorb complex fats or the fat soluble vitamins such as vitamins A,D,E, and K.

Most of the key hormones produced by the body are manufactured from cholesterol. Vitally important adrenal hormones such as cortisol as well as the sex hormones and pituitary hormones are all manufactured from cholesterol.

Contrary to popular opinion, the major source of this vital compound known as cholesterol is our own bodies rather than our diet. Humans manufacture 80% to 90% of their cholesterol within their own cells. Almost all cells of the body have this capability although most of it occurs in the liver.

Now knowing and appreciating the crucial role of cholesterol to biological function and even life itself, you can understand why the body must be able to manufacture its own supply. Life would be too fragile and uncertain if we had to depend on an external source of supply of cholesterol to survive. It is also clear why egg yolks are ultra-rich in cholesterol. Unlike mammalian fetuses, whose blood supply, and thus cholesterol supply, is linked to the mother, birds and reptiles must develop and grow entirely dependent on the nutrients contained in the egg. Because cholesterol is one of the elements most essential for growth and development, it is therefore present in abundance in the egg yolk.

Cholesterol was first identified chemically in 1784 as the primary component of gallstones. The name came from the Greek words *chole* (bile) and *stereos* (solid)..Most people tend to think of cholesterol as a fatty substance, but cholesterol is not a fat, but a sterol. What fats and cholesterol have in common is that they are fat soluble and thus both are listed under the general term "lipid" which is an operational term applied to all molecules that are fat soluble.

All biochemical compounds are either water soluble or fat soluble. Some may be water soluble at one end and fat soluble at the other. Water soluble substances such as salts and sugars will dissolve readily in water-based liquids and thus can be carried easily in the blood. Fat soluble substances, however, are impervious to water and tend to repel water molecules. They will dissolve only in certain solvents such as alcohol, ether, or chloroform. Fat soluble substances such as cholesterol and fats cannot dissolve in the water-based blood stream and therefore must be carried inside water soluble molecular complexes known as lipoproteins. Some have used the analogy of little lipoprotein "boats" carrying the fats and cholesterol as passengers in the blood. In recent years much has been written and discussed about the different lipoprotein "fractions" in the blood. The three most important of these are very low density lipoproteins (VLDL), low density lipoproteins (LDL), and high density lipoproteins (HDL). Discussions of atherosclerosis and coronary heart disease have dealt almost exclusively with the latter two—often referred to as "bad" cholesterol and "good" cholesterol respectively. In reality the only difference is in the lipoprotein, the carrier. The cholesterol is the same in both LDL and HDL and the notion that one is "bad" and the other "good" is nonsense. We will discuss the LDL/HDL evidence in more depth later.

The sum of all the cholesterol carried in the various lipoprotein fractions is called the total cholesterol. This is the level that most people are referring to when they discuss their cholesterol level. For more than 30 years the normal range for total cholesterol in virtually all testing laboratories was 150-350 milligrams per deciliter (mg/dl). Over the past 20 years the upper limit of what is considered to be normal or desirable has been ratcheted down;first to 300, then 260, 240, and now 200 mg/dl. These changes were not based on any scientifically compelling evidence but rather on the whims of a small group of anti-cholesterol proponents. The numbers are supposedly based on the results of a large study called the MR.FIT trial[1] (which we will examine in some detail later). But the data presented in that study showed only a 0.13% difference in CHD mortality between those with the lowest cholesterol levels (<182 mg/dl) and those with the highest (>244 mg/dl). That's not thirteen percent; it's thirteen *one hundredths* of one percent. This miniscule difference hardly seems to justify lowering the "normal" or "desirable" levels of cholesterol to levels that create a medical "problem" for half of the healthy population.

So how did cholesterol, a compound absolutely essential to life itself, come to be regarded as evil and toxic? Why did it become thought of as a major cause of atherosclerosis and coronary heart disease? How did the idea that diet was an important factor come into being? Unfortunately the results of some early experiments got researchers and theorists started on the wrong track. To understand how the current Cholesterol Theory evolved, it is necessary to go back about 140 years.

Knowledge about atherosclerosis and coronary heart disease was very scant in the 19th century. In the 1870s a German pathologist named Rudolph Virchow examined the plaques from arteries in patients who died and found that many contained significant amounts of cholesterol. He then conceived the initial version of the Lipid Hypothesis. He called the process lipid insudation because he felt that the cholesterol infiltrated the walls of the arteries directly from the blood and caused the AS he found there.

In 1912 another investigator produced cholesterol plaques in rabbits by feeding them an extremely high-cholesterol diet. At this point it was thought that all cholesterol came from the diet and it was thus reasonable to suppose that a diet rich in cholesterol could indeed be the cause of AS.

In 1925, however, it was found that the body manufactured most of its own cholesterol and that in fact, the body manufactured several times more cholesterol than was consumed in the diet. This discovery would eventually cause some to question the Lipid Hypothesis. But a number of investigators were convinced that diet was important and they played a great role in the further development of the Cholesterol Theory. This further evolution of the theory will be the main subject of the next Chapter, but, first, it will be useful to discuss why and how some of the early research led people astray.

Most people (and many doctors) have a seriously mistaken impression of how the process of atherosclerosis takes place. They imagine that excess cholesterol in the blood is deposited on the inner wall of the artery and, over time, builds up to a point where it begins to obstruct the flow of blood. Some have called this the clogged pipe model. Nothing could be further from the truth.

As mentioned in the previous chapter, plaques in the arterial wall are initiated by a proliferation of cells that form a dense fibrous cap. These are smooth muscle cells derived from the middle layer of the artery. Something triggers these cells to migrate inward and begin forming a proliferative plaque. A better analogy than the clogged pipe might be the formation of a callous. We all know when certain spots on the hand or foot are repetitively rubbed or irritated, the skin throws up a protective barrier by in the form of a callous. It may be that the trigger mechanism in plaque formation is a localized area of physical stress on the arterial wall and that the proliferative plaque is a protective/reparative process. Following the initial cellular proliferative phase of plaque formation, one may begin to see evidence of cholesterol inside the plaque. However, this is a variable process, giving some plaques with a large amount of cholesterol but also many with little or no cholesterol at all. The origin of the cholesterol contained in plaques is, of course, hotly debated, but there is some evidence to suggest that it may be a breakdown product from degenerating cells within the plaque.

In fact, the popular misconception about cholesterol deposits building into a plaque is only true in the animal feeding experiments mentioned earlier. First rabbits and then chickens were fed virtually pure cholesterol, which ran their cholesterol levels up into the 1000–2000 mg/dl range. When the animals' arteries were examined, they showed significant deposits of cholesterol. Cholesterol deposits were also found throughout most of the animals' bodies and vital organs. With the development of the electron microscope (not available to the early researchers) it was soon apparent that these cholesterol depositions were different from the plaques examined from human arteries. The cholesterol deposits in the arteries and vital organs of the animals are more characteristic of a lipid storage disorder that can be seen in a tiny percentage of people with rare genetic defects. In addition, these cholesterol depositions from the rabbits and chickens did not lead to the same complications as AS plaques in humans; they did not develop cracks or fissures and then progress on to heart attacks. When the cholesterol was removed from the diet, the deposits began to regress and disappear.

Rabbits and chickens are primarily herbivorous animals whose normal diet contains very little cholesterol. They do not have the same metabolic machinery to handle cholesterol as do the more carnivorous species. One might ask what would happen if humans were given large amounts of cholesterol in their diets. The answer is, not much. Humans are an omnivorous species and, except for a few with genetic defects, have all the necessary equipment to handle excesses. Back in the 1930s, numerous studies were done in which groups of people were given diets with 5–10 times the normal daily intake of cholesterol, usually in the form of several extra eggs per day. Although the cholesterol levels sometimes rose a little at first, they soon returned to very near their baseline levels. Other experiments in which cholesterol was almost completely eliminated from the diet showed similar results—cholesterol levels may have dipped a little at first but soon returned to the baseline. Rarely did any dietary change in cholesterol affect the blood cholesterol levels by more than a few percentage points.

The reason for this is that blood cholesterol levels are subject to a feedback-control mechanism. As mentioned earlier, we manufacture most of our own cholesterol and only a small percentage comes from the diet. It is through regulation of this manufacturing process that the blood cholesterol level is maintained despite dietary changes. Biology is replete with feedback-control mechanisms that govern the levels of many substances contained in the blood. Each individual has a range of blood cholesterol that is presumably set by the genes. When excess cholesterol is consumed, the body simply makes less. Conversely, if little or no cholesterol is consumed, the body simply steps up the rate of manufacture to restore the level to somewhere within the genetically set range.

It is important that I point out here that nobody disputes any of these facts. The medical literature and the nutritional journals contain dozens, and possibly hundreds, of articles on experiments documenting this mechanism and showing that diet has only a trivial effect on cholesterol levels, yet we are constantly exhorted (even nagged) about following "healthy" diets to lower our cholesterol. One might reasonably ask how anyone, in the face of near-unanimous contradictory evidence, could recommend such a diet with a straight face. It is a remarkable testament to the sheer stubbornness and talent for denial of the obvious that the adherents of the Cholesterol Theory cling to this fallacious concept.

A number of other features, statistics, and observations would also seem to contradict the Cholesterol Theory:

— CHD is predominantly a male disease, yet women on average have slightly higher cholesterol than men.. This is not to say that women do not suffer heart attacks, but men outnumber women somewhere between 5 to 1 and 10 to 1 in the incidence of true heart attacks (the statistics showing heart attack as the leading cause of death in women are based on death certificates which are notoriously unreliable as sources for medical statistics).

— There have been many documented cases of people with cholesterol levels ranging from 400 to 1000 mg/dl living to ripe old ages with never a hint of heart disease.

— Victims of heart attacks have cholesterol levels evenly distributed throughout the range of values. In fact, more than half of heart attack victims have cholesterol levels in the low normal range.

— Significant AS is normally not found in the veins or in the pulmonary arteries, where the pressures are much lower than in the systemic arteries. If the disease was due to a chemical substance in the circulation, one would expect it to affect all vessels equally. It is interesting that veins exposed to artery-level pressures such as those used in coronary bypass grafts or in the creation of arteriovenous fistulas for dialysis show the rapid development of AS, which was never present when the veins were performing their original functions.

— Atherosclerosis is a focal disease, meaning that plaques occur at various locations along the course of an artery, with relatively unaffected segments of artery between the plaques.

— Atherosclerosis does not occur at random locations. Rather, there is a pattern which can be predicted based on the distribution of physical stress on the inner portion of the arterial wall. There is a marked tendency for plaques to occur at branching points and along the lesser curvatures where the physical pressure forces are greatest.

— Atherosclerosis is not uniformly distributed throughout the body's various arterial systems. For example, advanced AS is commonly found in the arteries of the legs but very rarely in the arteries of the arms.

— Plaques are usually eccentric; that is, they occur on one side of the arterial wall rather than uniformly throughout the entire circumference of the arterial wall as one might expect with uniform exposure to a noxious chemical.

The above list is just a random assortment of observations that would seem to make the Cholesterol Theory counter-intuitive. Many more could be listed. It is reasonable to ask how the theory could evolve and gain general acceptance in the face of these anomalous facts. In order to understand this, we must go back to some of the original studies that came out of a branch of clinical science called epidemiology.

## CHAPTER FOUR

# HOW EPIDEMIOLOGY AND PHONY STATISTICS LED SCIENCE ASTRAY

*"Nothing so needs reforming as other people's habits."*

Mark Twain

Epidemiology is the study of common factors and patterns in the distribution of human diseases. Epidemiologists use statistical correlation to try to identify the causes of disease. As implied by the name, epidemiology was originally the study of epidemics and contributed greatly to improvement of human health by discovering sources of infectious diseases as well as environmental hazards such as impure water supply. Unfortunately, its methods have proven to be counterproductive when applied to chronic and/or degenerative diseases.

By the middle of the 20th century, the combined effects of antibiotics, vaccines, and routine public health measures such as chlorination of the water supply had pretty much eliminated infectious epidemics in the civilized world. Rejecting the options of graceful retirement or moving on to other fields of specialty, some epidemiologists began looking about for new worlds to conquer. Many felt that they could apply their techniques to the noninfectious diseases and identify the environmental factors they felt were causing those disorders that affect public health on a large scale—especially cancer and heart disease.

It was at this point that a momentous event occurred that would profoundly affect the nature of medical research for the next 50 years. In the mid-1950s, a team of British researchers led by Drs. Austin Hill and Richard Doll published a study linking lung cancer to cigarette smoking. Their survey of 60,000 British physicians showed a 24-fold increase in lung cancer among heavy smokers when compared to non-smokers. This was the first time an external agent was shown to be highly correlated with a serious disease.

It was also the **last** time. Despite more than 50 years of trying, epidemiologists have failed to identify a single factor that shows a correlation with any disease that even remotely approaches the degree of correlation between smoking and lung cancer. Unfortunately, this one early success stimulated a spate of unproductive epidemiological studies that continue to this day. The desperate attempts by hundreds of investigators to make their names by identifying their own "smoking guns" have generated lists of hundreds of "risk factors" for cancer and heart disease. Virtually none of these risk factors shows a level of correlation high enough to suggest the results are due to anything more than chance and/or bias.

Of course, even the high degree of correlation does not prove that cigarette smoking *causes* lung cancer. Obviously, it can't be "the cause," because many cases of lung cancer are known to occur in people who have never smoked. It may be that cigarette smoking activates or accelerates some process whose true cause was genetic or due to some other factor. For example, if we turn to a gardening analogy, a poorly nourished plant may thrive and produce blossoms or fruit when given a fertilizer, but that fertilizer was not the ultimate source of the flower or fruit.

Epidemiology is an observational science as opposed to an experimental one. The Hill-Doll smoking study is an example of an observational case-control study. In this type of study, a group of people afflicted with a certain disease or disorder is compared with a control group of people free of the disorder but otherwise similar in terms of age, sex distribution, and other demographic factors. The investigators examine the two groups, looking for differences in diet, lifestyle habits, or any other factor they feel may be involved in causing the disorder in question. The number of "risk factors" that can be examined in this way is virtually endless, limited only by the resources and imaginations of the investigators.

One problem with this type of study is that if enough factors are compared, one will find a number of correlations with the disease in question by chance alone. This is where the strength of the association or correlation becomes important. Most scientifically inclined epidemiologists will agree that a factor should not be considered to be even possibly significant unless the risk ratio is at least 3:1 or 4:1. That is, the percentage of those with the risk factor who have the disease should be 3 or 4 times the percentage of those without the risk factor who have the disease. For example, suppose one theorizes that having red hair is a risk factor for diabetes. If a control group of non-redheads is found to have a 10% incidence of diabetes, then 30%–40% of the redheads examined should show evidence of diabetes for this to even be *considered* as a possible risk factor.

A more serious problem with this sort of "risk factor" epidemiology has to do with the existence of confounding factors. Factors A and B may appear to be correlated with one another, but actually, both could be correlated with an independent third factor, C, so that A and B have nothing to do with each other directly. Here, C is the confounding factor. For example, a number of studies have attempted to link excessive alcohol consumption with the risk of developing cancer. Critics point out that people who drink heavily also are much more likely to smoke as well. It turns out that the smoking accounts for the increased cancer risk and that excessive alcohol consumption adds nothing further to the risk.

Because the cause of a disease or disorder under investigation is, by definition, almost always unknown, one can never be sure that there are not some unknown confounding factors giving a spurious credibility to the correlation between the factors being examined by the investigators. This alone should temper the enthusiasm of those who want to conflate statistical association or correlation into cause and effect.

Another fly in the epidemiological ointment has to do with the fundamental quality of the data being considered. Epidemiological studies seek to link a disease or disorder to the exposure to one or more risk factors. The difficulty often comes in trying to quantify that exposure. Often, a moment's reflection and the application of common sense to the analysis will show that the accuracy of measurement is open to serious question. For example, many studies in recent years have attempted to link all kinds of disorders to toxicity from radon gas. How can one measure past exposure to something like radon gas in the home and/or workplace? What about the figures given for dietary intake in the hundreds of studies seeking to link various disorders to certain foods or food groups? These provide detailed information on the diets of the participants, including daily caloric intake, percentage of saturated fats, unsaturated fats, protein, carbohydrates, etc. It sounds very impressive when they cite the benefit to group A from taking only 22% of their calories as saturated fats as opposed to group B's 29%; but where do these figures come from? Most studies use recall questionnaires, meaning the participants listed the foods they consumed during the prior 24 hours. Some questionnaires will use a one- or two-week period. Of course, participants must also be able to give the *quantity* of each food consumed. These data are then extrapolated back and said to represent the individual's diet over several years or, sometimes, entire lifetime. Aside from the obvious problem of fallibility of human memory, it has also been shown time and again that people tend to misrepresent their true food consumption so they appear less gluttonous or conform more closely to their perception of the investigator's idea of a "healthy" diet. These built-in errors are often referred to as "recall bias."

Confounding factors and biases of various types are ubiquitous problems in epidemiologic studies and are almost impossible to eradicate. They introduce systematic errors into any study where they may be present. This is an important distinction, because sophisticated statistical techniques as well as the calculation of confidence limits and "p" values are only applicable to random variation in the data. There is no way these statistical techniques can correct for systematic bias or error.

This brief discussion of the limitations of epidemiology should be sufficient to demonstrate that epidemiologic studies are worthless as providers of scientific proof. At best, epidemiologic studies only suggest areas of interest where true scientific investigation may be of value. At worst, they lead to blind alleys of research and thus squander tremendous amounts of money and scientific manpower that could have been more profitably employed elsewhere.

Nevertheless, the early evidence that gave impetus to the Cholesterol Theory and particularly the importance of diet came from epidemiologic studies.

One of the first influential studies was the Six Countries study,[1] published in 1953 by Dr. Ancel Keys. Dr. Keys was fairly certain that he knew the cause of the "epidemic" of coronary heart disease (CHD) in the United States—the American diet. Too much saturated fat and cholesterol in the diet was raising cholesterol levels in the blood and causing atherosclerosis (AS) and CHD. Dr. Keys set out to prove this by correlating the incidence of death from CHD with the amount of fat in the diet in several countries around the world. Indeed, he showed a nearly linear correlation between the percentage of fat in the diet and mortality from CHD in the six countries he selected.

When critically reviewing any scientific study, one must first determine the validity of the data. In the garbage-in–garbage-out (GIGO) model, inaccurate data renders all correlations and conclusions meaningless. In Dr. Keys' study, he correlated two different sets of data. One was the percentage of fat in the national diet, and the second was the death rate from CHD. Let's examine each of these in turn.

The national diet figures were derived from published international production rates of various foodstuffs minus the amount exported. The foods can be broken down into categories such as beef, poultry, dairy products, vegetables, and so on and, by estimating the percentage of fat in each, arrive at a figure for percentage fat in the "national diet." Obviously, this is going to be a rather gross estimate and there are a lot of potential sources of error.

For example, agricultural communities usually consume a large amount of their own produce. The foods in their diet may never show up in the international statistics. This alone will introduce significant error into the statistics for countries that have a lot of subsistence agriculture or a high percentage of small family farms.

What about your own personal diet? How consistent would it be from day to day, week to week, or year to year? How would it compare with that of your neighbors? How similar are the diets in, say, New Orleans and Kansas City? How about Miami, Florida, and Duluth, Minnesota? As one might imagine, the larger and more economically advanced countries will also have many more choices as well as abundance and diversity, thus rendering the concept of a "national" diet ludicrous.

For the sake of discussion, however, let's assume it is possible to derive a grossly accurate figure for "national diet." What about our second set of data—CHD mortality? These come from published national vital statistics, which, in turn, are almost entirely based on information taken from death certificates. It is vitally important to understand the limitations of death certificates as data sources because the inaccuracies in death certificates are enough to invalidate practically any study that uses them.

The death certificate is primarily a legal document. Its execution allows a decedent to be buried, the estate to be probated, and insurance to be paid. It was never intended to be a reliable source of medical data. The death certificate is typically filled out by the decedent's physician, who enters the cause of death to the best of his or her knowledge. The key phrase here is "to the best of his or her knowledge."

A typical scenario is that a patient, Mrs. Jones, is found dead in her home at age 95. Her physician really has no way of knowing how she actually died, but he has to enter a cause from an approved list of diagnostic codes called the International Classification of Diseases (ICD-9) for the certificate to be accepted. Causes such as "old age" or "natural causes" are not listed and are therefore not acceptable. If the physician does not fill out the certificate, Mrs. Jones becomes a coroner's case and her family has to wait for the bureaucratic wheels to turn before they can proceed with burial, probate, and the rest of their tasks; therefore, as a service to the family, the physician will usually enter a "default diagnosis." Typically, in this country we use CHD or an equivalent such as atherosclerotic heart disease because virtually every elderly person has some degree of AS and CHD. In other countries, different customs are followed and other "default diagnoses" used.

Naturally, the result of this process is that an inordinate number of elderly people who die of "old age" are counted as cardiac deaths. Of course, this causes a marked distortion in the statistical record and greatly inflates the national incidence of heart-related deaths. For example, one often hears or reads a statement such as "Heart attacks are the leading cause of death in women and exceed the combined death rates from all cancers." The vital statistics tables, however, show that the overwhelming majority of female CHD deaths occur after the age of 75; most are probably "diagnoses of convenience" as described for our hypothetical Mrs. Jones.

Consider a second, less common, scenario. A person collapses and dies suddenly or is found dead unexpectedly. Often, it's an apparently healthy person of middle age or beyond. Should the decedent be a celebrity or prominent public figure, the death will be reported in the media—invariably, as a heart attack, usually as a "massive heart attack." Although a detailed autopsy may be done to confirm cause of death for a prominent figure, this is rarely the case for the average person. The average decedent will usually go to a busy and overworked coroner's office that is primarily interested in making sure that the death was not due to criminal action.

This "sudden death syndrome" is another source of error in the heart attack statistics. Several studies have been done in which victims of sudden death have been subjected to detailed autopsies.[2] The autopsies show that about 1/3 of the deaths are due to heart attack, 1/3 are due to ruptured cerebral aneurysm or one of several other lethal disorders, and 1/3 have no obvious cause. Without the autopsy, almost all of these would have been signed out as cardiac deaths.

I can't resist interjecting my favorite death certificate anecdote, a true story concerning one of my senior partners who was called to a patient's home to pronounce the patient dead. He found the decedent lying in bed in peaceful repose and slid his stethoscope under the covers to listen for a heartbeat or any sound of respiration. Finding none, he returned to the office to await the arrival of the death certificate (usually brought to the office by the funeral home). Because the patient was past middle age and had a history of heart trouble, the doctor was, naturally, prepared to sign the patient out as a cardiac death. Imagine his surprise when the mortician called that afternoon and asked, "Doctor, are you aware that this man was shot in the chest?"

The bottom line is that mortality statistics on cause of death are unreliable and, therefore, virtually useless for scientific studies. One should keep this in mind when being told that "heart attack is the leading killer in the US," "heart attacks kill more women than all other diseases combined," or "disease X kills Y number of people per year in the US." Are any of these true? Who knows? The truth is that we don't have data accurate enough to know whether any of these or similar claims are true.

Most studies examining the accuracy of death certificates in the US have concluded that the error rate is 50% or more.[3] If this is true here, imagine how reliable the data are in less advanced countries where data collection is incomplete and many people have virtually no contact with the medical system.

Let's now return to Dr. Keys' study correlating cardiac death rates with high-fat diets. We can see the absurdity of drawing conclusions from correlations between two sets of inaccurate data. But let's again assume that the figures are roughly accurate for the sake of discussion, because, even granted such an assumption, his conclusions do not stand up when subjected to scientific analysis. Rather, they reveal a mindset and a method of reporting that are, unfortunately, all too common among the proponents of the Cholesterol Theory.

Critics of Dr. Keys' Six Country study point out that the same international statistics on foodstuffs and mortality were available for 22 countries at the time he did his research. Why did he not include all of these in his analysis? Because he chose the six that fit his theory and omitted the sixteen that didn't. Among these were countries with a low percentage of fat in their diets but high incidence of CHD death and vice-versa. This selective use of statistics to support a preconceived theory is not only unscientific but is dishonest. Unfortunately, it is also a common tactic employed by those who are more interested in pursuing an agenda rather than in finding the truth.

One of the omitted countries was France, where statistics showed a very high fat diet but a low CHD death rate. This is often referred to as "the French paradox" (paradoxical only to those who subscribe to the diet-heart connection). All kinds of ad hoc hypotheses have been advanced to explain this "paradox." The most popular was that drinking red wine conferred a protection against the deadly cardiac effects of the rich French diet. This was, of course, discussed and accepted without a scintilla of scientific evidence. In reality, the explanation is much simpler: The French mortality figures are no more accurate than those in the US or any other country. The difference is that in France, the "default diagnoses" on death certificates are myocarditis or hypertensive heart disease, rather than CHD. Therefore, the French statistics show a low incidence of CHD but an enormously higher incidence of myocarditis and hypertensive heart disease.

Findings that *support* the diet-heart connection can also be explained through a better understanding of the unreliability of the statistics. For example, Japan is one of the countries most often cited by the diet-heart enthusiasts because the Japanese have a low-fat diet and a low incidence of reported heart disease. But further analysis of the Japanese statistics shows that they have an enormously higher death rate from stroke than is recorded in the US. This seems puzzling because heart attacks and strokes are both the result of complications from underlying AS. As one might now guess, the answer lies in the way the death certificates are filled out. It turns out that in Japanese culture, death from a bad heart is very undesirable, but death from a brain disorder is more honorable and a sign of intelligence.

Incredibly, one still finds frequent references to Dr. Keys' studies in medical journal articles and reviews despite the fact that they have been shown to be textbook examples of how to lie with statistics. This type of study where published statistics are correlated with one another is often derisively referred to as "armchair research" or "number crunching."

Another type of epidemiological study—one that requires much more effort and planning—is called an observational cohort study. Here, a population is examined, tested, and subjected to various measurements and then followed over several years' time to see who develops the disease or condition under investigation.

Then the characteristics of the population that were measured and enumerated are examined to see if any correlate or "predict" the disease in question. In this way, so-called risk factors for the disease can be identified and, hopefully, suggest remediable causes, which can then be verified by scientific experiment. This latter statement about verification through scientific experiment is crucial because **correlation is not causation**. These last four words should be underlined four times and followed by multiple exclamation points, because most people (and especially the news media) don't seem to understand this fundamental truth. True causation can only be proven by experiments that rigidly adhere to the principles of scientific investigation and are reproducible. Epidemiology will not suffice.

# CHAPTER FIVE

# EPIDEMIOLOGY REDUX

*"Science is the great antidote to the poison of enthusiasm and superstition."*

Adam Smith

The best known and most influential observational cohort study on heart disease was initiated in the late 1940s in the town of Framingham, Massachusetts and, therefore, is known as the Framingham study. It virtually gave birth to the "risk factor" hypothesis of which the Cholesterol Theory is a subset. Unlike Keys' Six Country Study, which focused on dietary fats, Framingham specifically indicted cholesterol as a chief culprit in the causation of coronary heart disease.

In the late 1940s, the National Heart Lung and Blood Institute (NHLBI) decided to fund a study to determine the causal factors in coronary heart disease (CHD). A team of researchers from Boston University chose the small town of Framingham to provide the subjects for this study. The aim was to recruit as many healthy people between the ages of 30 and 62 as possible. These people would undergo physical examination and fill out detailed questionnaires regarding their diet, exercise patterns, smoking habits, and so on. These examinations would be repeated every two years. Also, it would be recorded when someone died or showed evidence of CHD, such as symptoms of chest pain, occurrence of nonfatal myocardial infarction (NFMI), or any sudden death that had no other apparent cause.

The study was begun in 1948 and continues to this day, although almost all of the original enrollees have died. Several reports have been published at different intervals during this time. After more than 20 years, analysis of the data have shown what were felt by the investigators to be significant correlations between several risk factors and CHD. These factors included being male, smoking cigarettes, having high blood pressure, and having elevated serum cholesterol.

In the previous chapter, we examined the importance of accurate data to generating reliable conclusions. We saw that the figures boldly advanced as percentage of fat in "national" diets are really only crude approximations. In the Framingham study as well as the other major studies cited as proof of the Cholesterol Theory the critical factor being investigated was the level of cholesterol in the blood. How accurate are these numbers?

In 1985, the College of American Pathologists sent test samples with cholesterol levels of precisely 263 mg/dl to 5,000 laboratories around the country.[1] The labs ran their usual cholesterol tests on the test sample and returned their results to the investigators. The measurements returned ranged from 197 to 397 although the majority were clustered between 222 and 294 mg/dl. In other words, a 10%–15% error was fairly common. Although improvements in lab techniques have since increased the reliability of cholesterol measurement, it must be kept in mind that all the epidemiologic and large cohort studies cited as proof of the Cholesterol Theory were carried out during a time when the measurement was of questionable accuracy. Moreover, the largest studies were collaborative efforts involving many different research centers and laboratories, thus compounding the problem of measurement error. But as we did with the dietary data, let's assume that the cholesterol measurements were accurate and reproducible. How did these measurements correlate with the end points chosen for the Framingham study?

The correlation of serum cholesterol level with CHD was rather weak. A perfect correlation between two measures would yield a correlation coefficient of 1.0. The correlation coefficient for cholesterol and CHD in the Framingham study was 0.36. Scientists generally like to see a value twice this high or more before even considering a causal relationship between two things.

Interestingly, the relationship was significant for men under 50 years old but not for men over 50, nor for women of any age. It would certainly be legitimate to question why a causative factor would not affect people equally regardless of sex or age.

Another fascinating result from this study was that diet showed no correlation with serum cholesterol or CHD. The investigators were unable to show any connection between high-cholesterol and/or high-fat diets with either blood cholesterol levels or any manifestation of CHD. Equally interesting is that this finding never appeared in any of the journal articles reporting the results of the study; rather, it was buried in a "technical"report filed by one of the authors in 1970.[2] This is another example of selective reporting by the anti-fat and -cholesterol forces who love to ignore data or studies that contradict their theories.

As mentioned in the previous chapter, there is a natural tendency among most people to consider correlation or association as causation, but scientists and researchers should know better.. There are a number of reasons why correlation may have nothing to do with cause and effect. For example, CHD and many types of cancer are diseases that occur with increasing frequency as we get older. Because people in economically advanced societies live longer than those in relatively poorer or more primitive societies, we would expect to see more of these diseases in economically advanced societies. Dr Eliot Corday addressed this point in an editorial in the *American Journal of Cardiology* in 1975.[3] Having just returned from a trip to China, he wrote:

> The late Isadore Snapper had taught us that in 1940 atherosclerosis was not a clinical problem in China because the Chinese ate a non-atherogenic diet. We now learn that there is a high incidence of coronary disease. When we asked our hosts what happened, they explained that the type of diet has not changed, but that life expectancy was less than 33 years at the time Snapper lived in China and now the population survives to an average age of 56.

Another differentiating factor between advanced and primitive societies is diet. The populations of more prosperous countries consume a larger proportion of protein and animal fats in their diets; thus, we should not be surprised if dietary factors do show a correlation with these diseases that are more prevalent in more economically advanced societies because of increased longevity. However, one can show even higher degrees of correlation for almost any other factor that distinguishes a prosperous society from a relatively poorer one. For example, some statistical studies have shown significant correlation between CHD and number of TV antennas or number of automobiles per capita, to name only two markers of societal prosperity.

My personal favorite is a study published by an Australian investigator in 1987.[4] He correlated the incidence of deaths due to automobile accidents with CHD mortality in Australia over a period of 25 years. He found that the correlation for men was 0.85 and for women 0.83, both of which are considerably higher than the coefficients reported for the more commonly cited associations such as cholesterol levels and dietary fat intakes. He also reported that the accident deaths showed a correlation coefficient of 0.98 with gasoline consumption and, thus, presumably the number of miles traveled by automobile. His conclusion was that these findings "must surely indicate that CHD could be a resultant effect of traveling in a motor vehicle." He didn't carry the analysis any further but could have just as reasonably concluded that the act of buying gasoline was what caused the CHD.

Because CHD incidence increases with age, one can show correlation of CHD with almost anything else that comes with age. For example, we can probably assume (without spending millions of dollars for a study) that having gray hair will correlate statistically with CHD and thus is a "risk factor," but this doesn't mean that dyeing your hair will be a realistic preventive measure.

Some people theorize that "stress" causes CHD. Although stress is subjective and impossible to quantify, we do know that the body reacts to psychologically perceived stress with increased production of cortisol—the so-called stress hormone. Because cortisol is manufactured from cholesterol, it may be that stress calls forth the manufacture of more cholesterol to ultimately produce more cortisol. Thus, if stress is the cause of CHD, cholesterol might just be an innocent bystander. In other words, stress may be a confounding factor causing both the heart disease and the higher cholesterol and these latter two have nothing to do directly. with one another.

Another possibility when two entities are correlated is that the postulated causation is backward—that is, the theory is that A causes B, but in reality, B causes A. Another hypothetical scenario may illustrate this cause-and-effect reversal: Many researchers feel that the atherosclerotic plaque may be the result of a repair mechanism for damage to the endothelial lining of arteries. Because the primary process in plaque formation is the proliferation of cells to form a cap, many new cells must be created to repair the damage. Because cholesterol is such a key component of cell membranes and other structures, this reparative process may elicit greatly increased cholesterol production to accomplish the necessary healing. In this scenario, cholesterol is not the cause of the plaque but a necessary result. The suppression of cholesterol production with drugs might, therefore, actually be harmful.

Even the most ardent epidemiologist will admit that correlation does not mean causation. They will agree that correlations can only suggest possible avenues for further study and that proof requires experiments based on the accepted principles of the scientific method. In the medical field, this means randomized clinical trials.

One would think that the lack of dietary association and the weak correlation with cholesterol and other modifiable risk factors would have dulled the enthusiasm of the anti-cholesterol crowd; however, they had the bit in their teeth. Ignoring the negative dietary data from Framingham and other studies and describing the cholesterol correlation as "strong" or "robust" in the face of obviously weak data, they were determined to press on to the next step—large and expensive (but taxpayer-funded) clinical trials.

## CHAPTER SIX

# THE EARLY CLINICAL TRIALS

*"Truth. . . never comes into the world but like a bastard, to the ignominy of him that brought her forth."*
John Milton.

There had been a few previous clinical trials that sought to investigate correlations between cholesterol and other factors with the incidence of coronary heart disease (CHD) but they were what are known as secondary prevention studies. That is, they used conventional scientific methodology to test the therapeutic efficacy of various drugs in patients with known heart disease. The purpose in the secondary prevention studies was not to prevent the disease but to head off future heart attacks in people at high risk because they had already suffered heart attacks in the past.

The structure of a randomized clinical trial is relatively straightforward. A sample is selected from a defined population, and the subjects are randomly assigned to treatment or control groups. The treatment may be a medication, surgery, a smoking cessation program, or any number of things. The control group receives either no treatment or a placebo. Placebos are used mostly when the treatment is a medication and a sugar pill, the placebo, is made up to look just like the treatment medication. Placebo-like control is obviously much more difficult when the treatment is surgery or counseling although there have been a few studies in which "sham" surgery was performed. The advantage of placebo use in drug trials is that the trials can be double-blinded. That is, through use of a third party, neither the subjects nor the researchers know who is getting the real medication or who is getting the placebo. This double-blinding is an ideal to strive for in scientific studies because it reduces the possibility of bias in reporting or interpreting results.

In clinical trials, the treatment and control groups take the medication or other intervention being studied for a period of time that is stipulated prior to the onset of the experiment. The defined end points (outcomes) are also delineated prior to the trial, monitored throughout the trial duration, and totaled at the conclusion. For cholesterol and CHD studies, the end points are almost always total mortality (all causes), CHD mortality, and nonfatal MIs (NFMIs)—that is, how many died from all causes, how many died from heart attacks, and how many suffered but survived heart attacks.

The largest and best known of the secondary prevention trials was the Coronary Drug Project.[1] This study took approximately 8000 males who had each had a prior heart attack (MI) and divided them into several groups. Five of the groups had about 1000 members each and were given four different drugs (two groups received different doses of the same drug). The remaining 3000 formed the control group and received placebo drugs. Two groups received estrogen hormone in two different dosages, one got thyroid hormone, another received clofibrate, and the last got niacin. Estrogen was tested on the theory that it might be the protective factor that explained the relatively low incidence of CHD in women. Thyroid hormone, clofibrate, and niacin were given because all work to lower cholesterol levels by different mechanisms.

So the 8000+ middle-aged volunteers who had all experienced a prior heart attack were randomly assigned to one of the five drug treatment groups or to the control group. The plan was to monitor these men for about seven years and see who died and who had further MIs. Unfortunately, the drug treatment for three of the groups had to be abandoned less than halfway through the planned seven-year period. So many excess deaths were occurring in the groups receiving the thyroid hormone and the doses of estrogen that the blinding had to be broken and these treatments stopped. One would think that this would raise serious questions about the theory that estrogen was the protective factor against CHD in women. To this day, however, one still hears "protection from heart disease" listed as one of the reasons for estrogen treatment for postmenopausal women. The two groups receiving the cholesterol-lowering drugs—niacin and clofibrate—showed no significant difference from the control group in CHD deaths or total mortality.

Undeterred by the negative findings, the Cholesterol Theory proponents argued, in effect, that perhaps treatment was too late for these men who already had established CHD. Interestingly, however, they continued to recommend treatment for this population. What was really needed, they said, was to test the effectiveness of cholesterol reduction in preventing the development of CHD in healthy people. This is called primary prevention. Experiments testing this hypothesis are known as primary prevention trials.

Because the anti-cholesterol forces were basically running the NHLBI and the American Heart Association (AHA), they had no problem getting funding to initiate the first large-scale primary prevention trial.

Some logistical problems occur in primary prevention trials that do not occur as much or to the same degree in secondary prevention studies. Because primary prevention trials deal with an apparently healthy population, the incidence of defined end points or outcomes such as CHD death, NFMI, and total mortality is going to be much less than that seen in a population with established heart disease, as in secondary prevention studies. Large numbers of subjects are therefore needed, so it makes sense to select those who are, theoretically, at highest risk for development of CHD to get the highest yield of "outcomes." Because dietary changes were known to have little, if any, impact on cholesterol or CHD, it was decided that other treatable risk factors should be treated as well. This approach had the additional advantage of more closely resembling what physicians were being told they must do in their treatment of their own patients.

The result of all this planning was the Multiple Risk Factor Intervention Trial,[2] which became known by the catchy title MR. FIT. This was a cooperative study carried out by 28 regional medical centers across the country and spanning a ten-year period between 1972 and 1982.

More than 360,000 healthy middle-aged men were screened for CHD risk using a risk factor equation developed by the Framingham researchers. The 12,000+ men with the highest risk scores were selected for the study. Most had high cholesterol levels, about 2/3 had significantly elevated blood pressure, and about 2/3 were cigarette smokers.

These MR. FIT subjects were randomly assigned to one of two groups. The treatment group was designated the Special Intervention (SI) group. The control group was called the Usual Care (UC) group. The "treatments" for the SI group were directed at reducing cholesterol through modifying diet, quitting or greatly reducing cigarette smoking, and controlling high blood pressure.

To achieve these ends, the members of the SI group and their families were given intensive instruction in picking out and preparing foods in a diet that was low in cholesterol, low in saturated fat, and high in polyunsaturated fat. They were instructed to keep detailed food diaries and met regularly with dietary consultants to review their progress. The smokers were subjected to a vigorous anti-smoking campaign with frequent counseling by doctors, psychologists, and other anti-smoking professionals. They reported every few months for blood testing, which would tell whether or not they were still smoking. Some underwent hypnosis or other therapies targeting their smoking habit. High blood pressure was treated aggressively, and overweight subjects were counseled by dieticians and others on weight-loss techniques and programs.

The UC group simply remained under the care of their own private physicians. They returned annually to the regional center for blood testing, blood pressure check, and questioning about their dietary patterns.

By almost any standard, this mammoth effort to lower risk factor levels through modification of lifestyle habits and blood pressure control was an enormous success. With the intensive dietary counseling, the SI group cut their cholesterol intake by more than 40%, saturated fat by almost 30%, and total calories by more than 20%. They increased their consumption of polyunsaturated fats by about 33%. The diet of the UC group was virtually unchanged.

In the SI group, the average reduction in blood cholesterol level was only about 7% despite these major dietary modifications. Interestingly, the cholesterol level in the UC group declined by 4%–5% leaving only about a 2% net reduction in the SI group.

Almost half the smokers in the SI group quit smoking, and blood pressure levels were lowered significantly. Thus, the MR. FIT study demonstrated that it is possible to modify some of the most important risk factors for CHD if enough time, money, and personnel are devoted to that task. The reported cost of this study was well over 100 million (taxpayer) dollars.

So what did we get with all this time, effort, and money? At the end of the study period, there had been 115 deaths ascribed to CHD in the SI group and 124 in the UC group. Total mortality (all causes) was 265 in the SI group and 260 in the

UC group. Obviously, neither difference is significant, even by the rather lax standard of "statistically significant" that is employed in so many medical journal reports.

One would think that the futility of risk-factor modification demonstrated here would be the final nail in the coffin of the risk factor concept.. One would think that even the most zealous dietary "nut" could not seriously recommend dietary change given the dismal results obtained here, but one would be wrong.

## CHAPTER SEVEN

# THE "DEFINITIVE" PROOFS

*"It is impossible for a man to learn what he thinks he already knows."*

Epictetus

The proponents of the Cholesterol Theory pointed out that there was only a net 2% difference in the cholesterol levels of the two groups in the MR. FIT study and that a much greater reduction would be necessary to show a benefit in the short term. This greater reduction would require drug therapy because dietary change was clearly inadequate (yet still highly recommended for one and all).

Fortunately, such a study was running almost concurrently with the MR. FIT trial. This was called the Lipid Research Clinics Coronary Primary Prevention Trial (LRCCPPT)[1] because it was carried out by a number of lipid research clinics that had been established around the country and funded by the National Heart, Lung, and Blood Institute (NHLBI). The publication of this study brought great joy to the hearts of the anti-cholesterol camp. "Eureka, we have proved it!" was the cry heard far and wide when its results were published in 1984. The "it" was the Cholesterol Theory.

It is almost impossible to overstate the importance that the cholesterol theorists attach to the LRC-CPPT study. They felt that they were literally tap-dancing on the graves of the critics of their beloved theory. The LRC-CPPT study has become the linchpin and the "final proof" of the lipid hypothesis. All published reviews and textbooks refer back to this as the bedrock of the proof that cholesterol is a major causative agent in coronary heart disease (CHD) and that the reduction of cholesterol will substantially reduce the risk of developing CHD. The introductory remarks in the published report state (for the first time) that all previous studies had been inconclusive. (Of course, one could equally well say that these previous studies conclusively proved that the Cholesterol Theory was hogwash.)

Because of the importance attached to this study, it is vital that we examine it in great detail. But before doing that, let's return briefly to a previous topic—end points in medical studies—and expound a little more on the subject.

End points, or outcomes, can be either "hard" or "soft." For example, total (all cause) mortality is a hard end point. Death is fairly easy to verify, and measurement of its incidence in a defined population is precise. CHD mortality, on the other hand, is a relatively soft end point. For all the reasons discussed previously, the diagnosis of death due to heart disease is frequently in error and is, therefore, a relatively unreliable statistic.

The other most commonly used end point in cardiac studies is the incidence of nonfatal myocardial infarction (NFMI). At first blush, this would seem to be a fairly firm and reliable end point because the definition of MI is explicitly spelled out and subject to verification by blood tests and electrocardiograms; however, studies designed to investigate the accuracy of MI diagnosis show otherwise.[2] Comparisons of autopsy diagnosis to clinical diagnosis show an average error rate of about 30%. These autopsy studies were not done by county coroners or lower-echelon community hospitals; rather, they were carried out at leading hospitals often affiliated with top teaching programs. If the degree of error is 30% for the "best and the brightest," what might it be for those of lesser ability or stature? The incidence of NFMI must therefore be considered a soft end point.

Other end points seen in cardiac studies are symptom related. They include frequency of chest pain, changes in exercise tolerance, and others. These end points are all subjective and, therefore, the softest of all.

In recent years, we have seen the emergence of "surrogate" end points. The most popular of these is "regression of coronary AS," where serial angiograms supposedly show lesser degrees of obstruction in patients taking cholesterol-lowering drugs. These differences in obstruction, however, are quite small and subject to measurement error. Furthermore, as discussed previously, the size of the obstructing lesion has virtually nothing to do with the physical changes (cracking or fissuring) that lead to MI and death.

The point of all this is that one must pay particular attention to the end points when evaluating any study or experiment. The only hard and reliable outcome is total mortality; therefore, total mortality should always be given the greatest weight. The soft end points are so subjective or prone to error that they should be given very little weight. The use of death certificate diagnoses is, in and of itself, sufficient cause to question the conclusion of any study that employs it. The usual response to this criticism of death certificate data (and other soft end points) is that "this is all we have." This, of course, merely confirms the lack of scientific rigor in the thinking of those who quote such studies as scientific evidence.

The other argument for accepting these soft end points is that large numbers will tend to even out the errors in measurement. Although this is statistically true, it is irrelevant to the CHD studies we are examining. These studies may show large numbers up front in the number of people screened and/or accepted into any given study, but the relevant numbers are those showing how many participants suffer the outcomes under investigation, and those numbers are never large.

With these points in mind, let's return to our analysis of the landmark LRC-CPPT study.

Because this was to be a primary prevention study, it would, like the MR. FIT trial, require a large number of subjects at the high end of the risk range for CHD. Almost half a million middle-aged men were screened, and a sample of 3,816 were selected for the study. These were the men with the highest cholesterol levels, which put them in the top 1% nationally in terms of cholesterol levels.. Even though women and 99% of men were excluded from the study, the authors and the rest of the anti-cholesterol crowd had no problem recommending that the results be extrapolated to include the entire population (including children).

These men were randomly assigned to a treatment or control group. The treatment group was given cholestyramine, a bile sequestrant resin which leeches cholesterol out of the system by binding with bile salts in the bowel and reducing their reabsorption. The recommended dose was six packets per day. Unfortunately, cholestyramine causes an inordinate amount of gastrointestinal side effects such as heartburn, gas, bloating, and constipation, so most patients couldn't tolerate the full daily dose. More importantly, a high incidence of obvious side effects seriously compromises the double-blinding because it is most likely that those participants suffering the most pronounced side effects are taking the experimental medication rather than the placebo. This loss of blinding eliminates one of the most important safeguards against bias in a scientific study.

Scientific studies require a written protocol outlining how the subjects will be selected and assigned to groups, how the data will be collected and the statistics analyzed, what the end-points will be and how they are defined, and so on.. The investigators in the LRC-CPPT study expected a cholesterol reduction of 25%. The primary end point would be the combination of CHD deaths and NFMIs. Other end points would be all-cause mortality and symptoms suggesting stroke and peripheral vascular disease. The researchers also set a high standard for statistical significance, stating that they would accept only a $p<0.01$ rather than the usual $p<0.05$. In the protocol outlining the plan for the study, the authors stated, "Since the time, magnitude, and cost of the study make it unlikely that it could ever be repeated, it was essential to be sure that any observed beneficial effect of cholesterol-lowering was a real one. Therefore…[significance] was set at 0.01 rather than the usual 0.05." [3]

This p value is an expression of statistical probability. Knowing its exact derivation is not important for our purposes now, but it roughly means the probability that the experimental result obtained could be a chance occurrence. Thus, $p < 0.05$ means that the likelihood that the given result was due to chance is less than 5%. A p value $< 0.01$ means that the likelihood of the result being due to chance is less than 1%. There is considerable debate over the true significance of a given p value, but that is not relevant to this discussion. I mention it here only because that was the criterion given before the trial began and, as we shall see, was later changed.

The LRC-CPPT study was carried out over a ten-year period. The authors reporting the results of the study in the *Journal of the American Medical Association (JAMA)* were pleased to report an unqualified success. Although cholesterol reduction was only about 8%, the investigators reported a 19% reduction in the primary end point—combined CHD deaths and NFMIs. The authors therefore claimed that each 1% reduction in cholesterol would give a 2% reduction in cardiac risk. It is important to know, however, that **the total (all-cause) mortality was essentially the same for both groups**. Because total mortality is the only true hard end point and the primary end point here was the sum of two relatively softer end points, we should examine the raw data to see what is really going on here.

The key data show 30 deaths from CHD plus 130 NFMIs in the treatment group, for a total of 160. This represents 7% of the 1906 subjects in the treatment group. The placebo group had 38 deaths from CHD plus 158 NFMIs, for a total of 196. This is 8.6% of the placebo group. Thus, the difference for the primary end point between the two groups is 8.6% minus 7.0%, which is 1.6%. So where does the figure of 19% come from? Divide 1.6 by 8.6, and you get about .19—in other words, 1.6 is about 19% of 8.6. The 1.6% difference is called the absolute risk reduction. The 19% figure is called the relative risk reduction. Both figures are technically correct. The absolute risk reduction gives a much more accurate picture of the true relationship, but the relative risk gives a more impressive-sounding number for those who are pushing their own theory.

How significant is the difference between 7.0% and 8.6%? Common sense tells us that this difference is of no practical significance. But what about the more esoteric criterion of statistical significance? According to the pretrial protocol, which called for a level of certainty with $p<0.01$, it didn't even come close. If one applies the more lenient criterion of $p<0.05$, it still fails the test when the typical two-tailed test is employed.

If one applies the $p<0.05$ criterion and uses the less rigorous one-tailed test, however, this difference barely qualifies as statistically significant. This is, in fact, what the investigators did. In one of the most flagrantly dishonest acts ever seen in a major medical study, the authors apparently changed the criteria for significance after reviewing the data.

This deception did not pass unnoticed and was subjected to a withering critique by Dr. Richard Kronmal in an article titled "Commentary on the Published Results of the Lipid Research Clinics Primary Prevention Trial" [4] published in *JAMA* a little more than a year after the study results were published.. There was no explanation given for why it took more than a year for the critique to be published, but knowing the power to suppress wielded by the proponents, we can hazard a few guesses.

In his critique, Dr Kronmal states:

> "The importance of the distinction between the one-sided and two-sided testing is that a much smaller relative difference between the two groups will be deemed statistically significant on the basis of a one-sided...than a two-sided test....The designers of the CPPT clearly recognized this fact in the article describing the design of the study....However, sometime between the design and the reporting of the results of the trial, the criteria that had been set up originally were changed....The critical aspect of this comment is not the P value that was set prior to the trial or the use of a one-sided test; it is that the observed beneficial effect of cholestyramine now has the characterization "statistically significant" (reported as $P<.05$) and that this is based on a change in criteria that apparently took place after analyzing the data."

On the question of the legitimacy of extrapolating results to groups not entered in the study, Dr. Kronmal states, "they… state that the results should be extrapolated to numerous population subgroups not included in this trial. Extrapolations should always be made with extreme caution, but in this instance the weak results should have dictated more caution than usual."

So, to put it bluntly, this "landmark" study, the "final proof" of the Cholesterol Theory, is based on a deceptive presentation of an insignificant statistical difference between the treatment and control groups. Whether scientific fraud also took place is certainly open to question.

Although the LRC study is most often cited as the keystone to the edifice of "proof" of the Cholesterol Theory, the proponents also frequently cite a second clinical trial as providing the confirmation of the "proof" given by the LRC study. This confirmatory study is known as the Helsinki Heart Study[5] because it was carried out by researchers in Helsinki, Finland.

The Helsinki Heart Study is a virtual clone of the LRC experiment. Like the LRC, this was a primary prevention trial whose subjects were healthy males between the ages of 40 and 55 and who were said to be at high risk for CHD because of their high blood cholesterol levels. About 19,000 men were screened; 4,081 with the highest cholesterol levels were selected for the study. The average cholesterol level for those selected was 289 mg/dl. The 4,081 men were randomized into treatment and control groups. The treatment group was given a drug called gemfibrozil, and the control group was given a placebo. The study was carried out for 5 years, although about 1/3 of the subjects dropped out during this time.

Gemfibrozil is closely related to the cholesterol-lowering drug clofibrate, one of the drugs used in the Coronary Drug Project described earlier. Gemfibrozil lowers total cholesterol and LDL cholesterol (the so-called bad cholesterol) but has the further effect of raising HDL (the so-called good cholesterol); thus, one would expect a considerably greater benefit in prevention of CHD with this drug because many theorists feel that raising the "good" cholesterol (HDL) is as least as important as if not more important than lowering the "bad" cholesterol (LDL).

In fact, the study subjects taking gemfibrozil initially raised their HDL levels about 15%, although this declined to a 10%–11% increase over time. Total cholesterol was reduced by about 11% and LDL cholesterol by about 10%.

So what were the results from taking this drug that delivered on its promise of "down with the bad" and "up with the good"? Table 7.1 summarizes the pertinent numbers.

TABLE 7.1   Helsinki Heart Study

| | Gemfibrozil | | Placebo | | Absolute Risk Reduction |
|---|---|---|---|---|---|
| | (n=2051) | | (n=2030) | | |
| | No | % | No | % | |
| NFMI | 45 | 2.2 | 71 | 3.5 | 1.3% |
| CHD Deaths | 11 | 0.5 | 13 | 0.6 | 0.1% |
| Combined NFMIs and CHD Deaths | 56 | 2.7 | 84 | 4.1 | 1.4% |
| Total Mortality | 45 | 2.2 | 42 | 2.1 | -0.1% |

The only hard end point (total mortality) shows more deaths in the drug group than the controls. Of course, the authors largely ignore this fact, remarking only that the difference is not statistically significant. Instead, they (like the LRC study did) chose to combine the two relatively soft end points of CHD deaths and NFMIs. These combined figures show an incidence of 2.7% in the treatment group and 4.1% in the control group. A difference of 1.4% wouldn't seem very significant even if the end points of CHD deaths and NFMIs were rigorously defined and free of diagnostic error, but attributing significance to a 1.4% difference between end points whose determinative error rate may be as high as 50% in a study where nearly 1/3 of the participants dropped out is taking statistical manipulation to new heights of absurdity.

.

Naturally, nowhere in the report do the authors mention a risk reduction of 1.4% (absolute risk); rather, they report a reduction of 34%. By now, you can probably tell that this is our old deceptive friend, relative risk (1.4 is 34% of 4.1).

Thus, the two largest and best-controlled prospective studies of cholesterol-lowering therapies show remarkably similar results. Most important, both showed no significant difference in the only truly hard end point—total mortality. Both showed trivial differences in the relatively soft end points, which are subject to considerable diagnostic error. Moreover, these trivial differences were deliberately presented in a deceptive form to give them a spurious credibility they do not deserve.

Some people would object that these studies were carried out more than twenty years ago and that, surely, there must have been others documenting the connections between diet, cholesterol, and heart disease. In fact, this is not true. As the Lipid Research Clinics investigators stated in their pre-study protocol, "the time, magnitude, and cost of the study make it unlikely that it could ever be repeated." And it never was repeated. There have been no further studies on the fundamental relationship between cholesterol and heart disease. Rather, the Cholesterol Theory was said to be proved by the two foundational studies cited above. All subsequent research has mostly involved empirical testing of various treatments and often employed surrogate end points.

The only possible exception to this is the Women's Health Initiative, which was published in *JAMA* in 2006. More than 40,000 women were followed for about 8 years to determine if a low-fat diet would reduce the incidence of CHD, stroke, colon cancer, or breast cancer. In a well-designed and -executed study, the authors showed that the low-fat diet had no effect on the incidence of any of these disorders. This was, of course, no great surprise, but the most interesting thing was the reaction of the researchers and others who seem to be emotionally wedded to the diet-health connection..

They almost uniformly expressed "disappointment" in the results of what was intended to be a landmark study, thus revealing their personal biases. Even more incredible, many said—in effect—that despite the results of this study, they still felt that a low-fat diet was important for good health.

In an ideal world where truth and justice prevail, critical review of these experiments would have sunk the Cholesterol Theory once and for all. But, as we have seen, the anti-fat and -cholesterol forces are nothing if not persistent, and no amount of contradictory data seems adequate to reject their theory.

Fortunately for them, at the time when the LRC-CPPT and Helsinki studies were completed  a whole new class of drugs was coming into development—a class that promised to dramatically lower cholesterol levels and thus provide the researchers with more fodder with which to conduct more multimillion-dollar studies at taxpayer expense.

## CHAPTER EIGHT

# STATIN DRUGS TO THE RESCUE

*"One of the first duties of the physician is to educate the masses not to take medicine."*

Sir William Osler

In 1987 a new drug called lovastatin (trade name Mevacor) was approved for use in lowering cholesterol. This was the first of a group of related drugs which are popularly known as statins. Within a short time, other pharmaceutical firms came into the market with their "copycat" statins such as pravastatin (Pravachol), atorvastatin (Lipitor), and simvastatin (Zocor). They all do essentially the same thing—reduce serum cholesterol by blocking the manufacture of cholesterol in the liver and other cells. What excited the anti-cholesterol forces was that these drugs lowered cholesterol by 30%–40 % and sometimes more. No more would they have to settle for piddling 5%–10% reductions in cholesterol, which yielded only equivocal clinical results in their experimental trials. Now they had weapons powerful enough to demonstrate the true value of serum cholesterol reduction.

To this end, several studies were carried out on different populations. The results of five of these studies are summarized in Table 8.1, but it's worth discussing each study and its design. The first three were secondary studies—in which the subjects had known preexisting coronary heart disease (CHD). The last two were primary studies, in which presumably healthy subjects had no prior history of CHD.

## TABLE 8.1. MAJOR STUDIES OF STATIN DRUGS

| Name of Study (Drug used) | Patient Population | Total Mortality (Drug/ Control) | CHD Mortality (Drug/ Control) | Nonfatal CHD (Drug/ Control) |
|---|---|---|---|---|
| 4S (simvastatin) | CHD-high cholesterol | | | |
| Absolute numbers | | 182/256 | 111/189 | 353/502 |
| Percentages | | 8.2/11.5 | 5.0/8.5 | 15.5/22.6 |
| CARE (pravastatin) | CHD-normal cholesterol | | | |
| Absolute numbers | | 180/196 | 96/119 | 135/173 |
| Percentages | | 8.6/9.4 | 4.6/5.7 | 6.5/8.3 |
| LIPID (pravastatin) | CHD-all levels cholesterol | | | |
| Absolute numbers | | 498/693 | 287/373 | 336/463 |
| Percentages | | 11.0/14.1 | 6.4/8.3 | 7.4/10.3 |
| WOSCOPS (pravastatin) | No CHD High cholesterol | | | |
| Absolute numbers | | 106/135 | 38/52 | 143/204 |
| Percentages | | 3.2/4.1 | 1.2/1.6 | 4.3/6.2 |
| AFCAPS (lovastatin) | No CHD Normal cholesterol | | | |
| Absolute numbers | | 80/77 | 11/15 | 116/183 |
| Percentages | | 2.4/2.3 | 0.33/0.45 | 3.5/5.5 |

The Scandinavian Simvastatin Survival Study (4S)[1] was carried out in a number of cooperating centers throughout the Scandinavian countries. More than 4,000 patients (80% male and 20% female) were randomized into drug-treatment and control groups. Only patients with high cholesterol were chosen for this study; mean cholesterol level was 263 mg/dl. After 5.4 years, the results showed modest improvement in all three end point categories—total mortality, CHD deaths, and nonfatal myocardial infarction (NFMI). Although the differences were hardly earthshaking, it was the first study ever to show some benefit in all three outcomes. But to hear the authors and the anti-cholesterol mob tell it, one would have thought they had discovered the Rosetta stone. Note that the differences get higher as the end points get "softer." Also, the improvement was seen in only the men. The women, who comprised 20% of the study population, showed no significant benefit.

The most interesting feature of this trial was not even mentioned in the published report. There was a total disconnection between the improved outcomes and both the initial cholesterol level and the degree of cholesterol lowering attained. In other words, protection against CHD was the same whether the initial cholesterol was high or low, and the degree of protection did not correlate with the degree of cholesterol lowering. Subjects whose cholesterol went down a relatively small amount benefited to the same degree as those whose cholesterol levels declined a lot. This disconnection is called "lack of normal exposure-response" and generally means that the factor under investigation is not the true cause of the disorder. In plain English, the small benefit conferred by the drug was not due to its effect on cholesterol but rather to some other cause.

Another secondary study was the Cholesterol and Recurrent Events Trial (CARE).[2] This experiment also involved about 4000 subjects who had a prior heart attack but normal cholesterol levels (defined as <240 mg/dl). The mean cholesterol level for the group was 209 mg/dl. The subjects were randomly assigned to either the treatment group, which received pravastatin, or a control group, who took a placebo. After five years, there were no significant differences in total mortality or CHD mortality. There was a slight reduction in NFMI, which barely achieved statistical significance.

The third secondary trial was the Long-term Intervention with Pravastain in Ischemic Disease (LIPID)[3] study. Approximately 9,000 subjects with prior CHD and with cholesterol values that covered the entire range were randomized between pravastatin and placebo groups. After six years of follow-up, there were small but statistically significant decreases in all three outcomes for the pravastatin group. The magnitude of the differences was similar to that seen in the 4S study.

The West of Scotland Coronary Prevention Study (WOSCOPS)[4] was a primary prevention trial that enrolled more than 6,000 healthy males with elevated serum cholesterol levels. The mean cholesterol level for the group was 272 mg/dl. Subjects were randomly assigned to either pravastatin or placebo. After 4.4 years, there were no significant differences in total mortality or CHD mortality. There was a slight reduction in NFMI in the pravastatin group.

The second of the primary prevention trials was the Air Force Coronary Atherosclerosis Prevention Study (AFCAPS).[5] Approximately 5,000 men and 1,000 women with normal cholesterol levels and no prior history of CHD were randomized to treatment with lovastatin or placebo. After 5.2 years there was no significant difference in total mortality or CHD mortality. There was a slight reduction in the combined end points of NFMI and chest pain in the group receiving lovastatin.

All of these studies exhibit certain similarities beyond their contrived names designed to give them catchy and memorable eponyms. Typically, they show little or no difference in total mortality and CHD mortality and only small differences in NFMI. At least three of the five studies had active participation in the planning and execution of the trial by employees of the pharmaceutical firm whose drug was used in the study. Most important, all the studies showed the same disconnection or lack of normal exposure-response that was described for the 4S trial. In other words, the small protective effect of the statin drugs against NFMI had nothing to do with their lowering of cholesterol. One observer was quoted as saying that "claiming that statins reduce the risk of heart disease by lowering cholesterol is like saying that aspirin reduces the risk of heart attack by reducing headaches." What a delicious irony that the final proof that cholesterol has nothing to do with CHD would come from trials of drugs specifically designed to lower cholesterol.

So what is it that the statin drugs do that provides this very modest degree of protection against heart attack? It turns out that these drugs have anti-thrombotic properties similar to aspirin and other anti-platelet drugs. That is, they inhibit the early phases of blood clot formation. In fact, studies using aspirin have shown an almost  identical degree of protection against NFMI as the statins.

The *British Medical Journal* reported a "Collaborative Overview of Randomized Trials of Anti-Platelet Therapy" in 1994.[6] They combined the results of 174 trials of anti-platelet therapy. Most of these experiments used low-dose aspirin, and the rest used other drugs that have essentially the same effect on platelet function in blood clotting as does aspirin. Unfortunately, these investigators didn't include a CHD mortality end point; they combined coronary deaths with those due to stroke and "deaths from unknown causes" into an end point they labeled "Vascular Death." The figures for this end point therefore can't be compared to the CHD mortality data from the other studies. The investigators did, however, use total mortality and incidence of NFMI as end points, and these can be directly compared with the results from the statin studies.

Tables 8.2 and 8.3 below compare the outcomes from the anti-platelet studies with those from the five statin studies described earlier for their comparable end points of total mortality and NFMI. These figures show that the small degree of "protection" afforded by the statins is really no better than that seen with low-dose aspirin.or comparable anti-platelet drugs.

.

Table 8.2. Total Mortality

|  | Drug | Control | Absolute Risk Reduction | Relative Risk Reduction |
|---|---|---|---|---|
| Statin trials | 6.6% | 8.2% | 1.6% | 19% |
| Anti-platelet Trials | 6.8% | 7.9% | 1.1% | 14% |

Table 8.3. Nonfatal Myocardial Infarction

|  | Drug | Control | Absolute Risk Reduction | Relative Risk Reduction |
|---|---|---|---|---|
| Statin trials | 7.5% | 10.5% | 3% | 29% |
| Anti-platelet Trials | 2.4% | 3.5% | 1.1% | 31% |

Another interesting study was published in the *American Journal of Epidemiology* in 2002. Titled "Water, Other Fluids, and Fatal Coronary Heart Disease,"[7] this study was part of a larger cohort study known as the Adventist Health Study. More than 20,000 men and women with no history of prior heart disease, stroke, or diabetes were enrolled. These people filled out detailed "lifestyle" question-naires regarding diet, fluid intake, smoking, exercise, and so on. They were fol-lowed for six years, and deaths from "fatal coronary heart disease" were recorded. The criteria for the diagnosis of "fatal CHD" were essentially the same as those used in the other studies discussed here and in the previous chapter.. This partic-ular report focused on the quantity of daily water intake and its relationship to subsequent fatal CHD. The investigators broke down the water intake into three groups. People consuming less than 2 eight-ounce glasses of water per day were the reference group. Those drinking 3–4 glasses daily or 5 or more glasses daily formed the other two groups, which were then compared to the reference group. Unfortunately, very little raw data is given in this report. Rather, the authors report their results only in terms of relative risk reduction, which, as we have seen earlier, is often grossly misleading. They probably chose to do this because the total CHD mortality for their subject population was only 1.2% and, therefore, the differences between the groups were probably only on the order of 0.1%–0.2%. Nevertheless, the relative risk reduction achieved with increased water consumption can be compared with that attained by statin drug therapy, as seen in Table 8.4 below.

Table 8.4. CHD Mortality

|  | Relative Risk Reduction |
| --- | --- |
| Statin Trials | 28% |
| 3–4 Glasses Daily | 44%* |
| >5 Glasses Daily | 52%* |

*Relative risk reduction compared to those drinking less than 2 eight-ounce glasses of water daily

Can one deduce from these reports that taking low-dose aspirin or drinking extra water will provide a significant degree of protection from heart attack? Absolutely not. These studies suffer from the same methodological problems as most of those cited before. But anyone who trumpets the virtues of statin drugs must acknowledge that the same "scientific" evidence shows that taking aspirin or increasing water consumption can accomplish the same quantitative result. Of course the cost of only a few days' therapy with statins would buy a year's supply of aspirin and drinking water. The other important difference is that the statins can have serious side effects—including death—whereas taking low-dose aspirin and/or drinking more water is virtually risk free.

The side effects of the statin drugs deserve a little more attention here because they have become the most prescribed drugs in the US. These side effects may be short term or long term. The short-term effects are generally well known, whereas the long-term effects are completely unknown but frightening in their possibilities.

The chief short-term side effects involve damage to the liver or the skeletal muscles. A number of patients have suffered severe liver damage from statin drugs, and some have died. This is why frequent blood tests must be taken to check the liver enzymes while a patient is taking any of these drugs. If the enzyme levels rise, then the drug must be stopped. The muscle damage that can result from statins is called rhabdomyolysis and involves massive destruction of skeletal muscle. The breakdown products from the muscles include a large load of protein, which can then affect the kidneys and cause them to fail. This is why patients are told to always tell their doctor about any symptoms of muscle weakness. The frequent blood tests required for patients taking statins also include measurements of muscle enzymes; elevation of these enzymes is also a mandate for discontinuation of the drug.

There have also been reports of neuropathic damage and cognitive dysfunction with memory loss caused by statins. However, these are disorders with a larger subjective component and can't be quantitatively demonstrated like the liver and muscle disorders.

As severe as some of these short-term side effects can be, they pale into relative insignificance when compared to the potential long-term problems. The chief difficulty here is that no one knows what the long-term effects may be from altering the basic biochemistry of the human body over a period of time. Because cholesterol is the key element in the formation of cell membranes, which are the protective coat for the cells, it may be that blocking cholesterol's production will weaken the protective barrier and allow the entry of toxins or carcinogens that were previously excluded. There are disturbing reports of increased cancer in some cholesterol-lowering studies, but, in fact, this process may take many years to play out. It's enough at this point to acknowledge that the long-term effects are completely unknown. This is a risk that should receive serious attention before half the population is placed on these drugs that, in effect, accomplish nothing more than low-dose aspirin or an extra glass or two of water each day.

# CHAPTER NINE

## THE CRITICS DISSENT

*"cynic n.: a blackguard whose faulty vision sees things as they are, not as they ought to be."*

Ambrose Bierce

We began this saga with the discovery of cholesterol in the atherosclerotic lesions of the arteries in the 1870s. Many would say that we've come a long way in the past 130 years. But have we really? What we have today is still Virchow's lipid insudation theory with a few added wrinkles and dressed up with some modern jargon.

The modern history of the Cholesterol Theory has its origin in the attempt by a group of well-intentioned researchers to identify "risk factors" for coronary heart disease (CHD). Despite repeated demonstrations that risk-factor modification has no effect on atherosclerosis (AS) or CHD, the theory is still alive and well today. The Cholesterol Theory, which is a subset of the Risk Factor Theory, was given credence by a group of investigators who were philosophically committed to the concept of lifestyle modification as a cure for the "epidemic" of CHD. They took some weak epidemiological evidence and conflated it into the modern

Cholesterol Theory and were able to parlay this into a multibillion-dollar research industry funded by the taxpayers. Through their control of the two major institutional structures, the American Heart Association (AHA) and the National Heart, Lung, and Blood Institute (NHLBI), they were able to effectively stifle dissent by refusing to fund research by those who disagreed with their theory. Because these institutions are also the chief conduits to the mass media, they have been able to propagandize the general public on the subjects of diet, cholesterol, and heart disease, successfully promoting a theory that has no credible scientific evidence behind it.

Lest the reader think that this is an unduly harsh view of these events by an isolated crank, permit me to quote George V. Mann, Sc.D. M.D. Professor of Biochemistry at Vanderbilt University School of Medicine. In an editorial printed in the *American Heart Journal* in 1978, he wrote:

> For 25 years the treatment dogma for coronary heart disease (CHD) has been a low cholesterol, low fat, polyunsaturated diet. This treatment grew out of a reasonable hypothesis raised in 1950 by Gofman and others, but soon a clot of aggressive industrialists, self-interested foundations, and selfish scientists turned this hypothesis into nutritional dogma which was widely impressed upon physicians and the general public. A nadir was reached when zealous doctors and salesmen arranged such "prudent" meals for national meetings of cardiologists, rather like Tupperware teas. There grew up in the interface between science and the

government funding agencies a club of devoted supporters of the dogma which controlled the funding of research, a group known by the cynics among us as the "heart mafia". Critics or disbelievers of the diet/heart dogma were seen as pariahs and they went unfunded, while such extravagancies as the Diet/Heart trial, the MRFIT trial and a dozen or more lavish Lipid Research Centers divided up the booty. For a generation, research on heart disease has been more political than scientific. All this resulted from the abuse of the scientific method. A valid hypothesis was raised, tested, and found untenable. But for selfish reasons, it has not been abandoned.

Some may wonder why certain researchers and institutions behave the way they do and promote a scientifically vacuous theory. Self-interest, careerism, and institutional imperatives may explain a lot of this, but why has practically the entire medical profession been taken in along with the general public? Why does the public accept these dictums that fly in the face of common sense and historical experience?

To answer these questions we must leave the realm of science and swim in the murkier waters of speculation, psychology, and human emotions.

## CHAPTER TEN

## WHAT KEEPS THE BIG LIE ALIVE

*"Nothing is easier than self-deceit. For what each man wishes, that he also believes to be true."*

Demosthenes

*"The masses have never thirsted for the truth. Whoever can supply them with illusions is easily their master; whoever attempts to destroy their illusions is always their victim."*

Gustave LeBon

In attempting to answer the questions posed at the end of the last chapter, we could benefit from breaking them down into categories and examining separately the motives and incentives facing the scientific investigators, the major institutional backers, the commercial interests, the medical profession, and, finally, the general public.

### The Investigators

Scientists are no different from anyone else. They become just as enamored with their own ideas and theories as the rest of us. Dr. George Mann illustrated this beautifully by quoting a 19th century philosopher who wrote:

The moment one has offered an original explanation for a phenomenon that seems satisfactory, that moment affection for his intellectual child springs into existence and as the explanation grows into a definite theory, his parental affections cluster about his offspring and it grows more and more dear to him...there springs up also unwittingly a pressing of the theory to make it fit the facts and a pressing of the facts to make them fit the theory.

The intensity with which many scientists defend their pet theories is comparable to that of a mother bear defending her cubs. In the past, heretics were hung or were burned at the stake; today, thankfully, they are allowed to live but are merely denied funding.

Consider the scientist who has spent 10–20 years or more researching a subject and has virtually built his career on a certain set of ideas or theories. It is, of course, extremely difficult for him to one day throw up his hands and say, "Well, I guess that was a waste of time." Rather, he will expend tremendous amounts of time and energy (and taxpayer dollars) trying to validate and justify his life's work.

Career incentives will also play a large role in determining the type of research that will be done. For example, some would maintain that the type of research needed to discover the true causes of atherosclerosis (AS) and coronary heart disease (CHD) involves basic laboratory research requiring knowledge of and familiarity with the techniques of histology, biochemistry, cellular biology, and other areas. But most medical research is carried out by M.D.s on the faculties of university medical schools.

Although some doctors think of themselves as scientists, they really aren't—at least not in the sense of those scientists capable of doing basic research. This is not a criticism, just a statement of fact. Doctors are trained in human anatomy and physiology and in how to apply this knowledge to the diagnosis and treatment of disease; they are not trained to do basic research. In spite of this, academic advancement is almost entirely based on the number of papers an individual can get published in the medical journals and on its corollary—how much research grant money one can bring to the university.

What is the academic doctor to do? Many solve the problem by cranking out useless epidemiologic studies in which they (or, more typically, assistants) collect survey data or published statistics, feed them into a computer, and generate statistical correlations. These "studies" are often real win-win-win situations for the doctor, the media, and the academic institution. The doctor gets a "scientific" paper published to add to his or her list of publications. The media, which love this sort of nonsense, get a dramatic headline or lead story for the week (for example, "Doctors today announced that they have learned that people who drink x cups of coffee per day have twice the normal incidence of y disease" or "In troubling news out of X University, doctors have found a link between cell phone use and brain cancer.") The academic institution gains in prestige with the publicity, which can only help in the institution's never-ending quest to attract "high profile" researchers who can bring in the big grant money.

.

## The Institutions

The incentives facing the institutions are inexorably tied in with those of the investigators because the hierarchies of the dominant institutions are almost entirely occupied by the same people whose careers and reputations are built around the Diet-Heart and Cholesterol Theories. The American Heart Association (AHA) and National Heart, Lung, and Blood Institute (NHLBI) are the two dominant institutions. Together, they administer over 90% of the grant money for cardiovascular research. Thus, any dissenters from the established dogma will find it almost impossible to get their research funded.

The chief imperative of any institution or organization is survival. To ensure their survival (and, hopefully, growth) they must both have a purpose and show that they are "doing something" to achieve that purpose.

The AHA is a private organization that has achieved a semi-official status in the eyes of most people as a spokesman for those in the cardiac related fields. Its chief purpose is to raise money to support research and disseminate information to the public on topics related to heart disease. In reality, it is sort of a medical analog to the chamber of commerce. Desperately in need of a cause to promote, the AHA took to the Diet-Heart Theory like a duck to water. Because any organization dependent on voluntary public support needs a cause with broad public appeal, the diet-heart nexus was ideal. And because food is a familiar commodity that everyone encounters daily and just about everybody thinks that what they eat is a major determinant of health, this was a cause that lots of people could get behind. The AHA could sponsor low-cholesterol food fairs, walks or runs to "combat heart disease," and a whole host of other fund-raising activities. Of course, it didn't hurt that the food companies would pay thousands of dollars to the AHA for the right to display the official AHA seal of approval on their food products.

Like the investigators whose careers and reputations are closely linked with the Cholesterol Theory, the AHA couldn't, after years of nagging people about their diets, suddenly change course and say, "Gee, there's no real evidence to support this idea we've been pushing. Sorry we wasted all that money you gave us."

The NHLBI is a government institution and thus will suffer from all the limitations inherent in a government bureaucracy. The imperatives to protect one's own turf, cover your rear end, and constantly try to expand the scope, personnel, and budget of your department or division will ensure that much more time and effort are expended on useless activities than productive pursuits. Of course, it also ensures that politics will play a major role. There is no surer sign of this than the fact that the NHLBI convened a "Consensus Conference" in 1984 to reach agreement on the answers to some key questions concerning cholesterol and CHD.

Consensus conferences are quite new to the world of science and inherently unscientific in their nature. Either a theory passes scientific muster or it doesn't. You can't vote it into existence by majority rule. The best formulation of this rather basic principle was expressed by the fiction author (and physician) Michael Crichton in his novel *State of Fear*:

Let's be clear; the work of science has nothing whatever to do with consensus. Consensus is the business of politics. Science, on the contrary, requires only one investigator who happens to be right which means that he or she has results that are verifiable by reference to the real world. In science, consensus is irrelevant. What is relevant is reproducible results. The greatest scientists in history are great precisely because they broke with the consensus. If it's consensus, it isn't science. If it's science, it isn't consensus. Period.

Just as randomization is a key element in a successful experiment, the selection of the participants is the key to a successful consensus conference. A smooth and pleasant conference is ensured by excluding troublemakers who might disagree with the preordained "consensus."

In a wonderful little opinion article titled "Nonsensus Consensus" published in the *Lancet*, Dr, Petr Skrabanek wrote:

> [T]he very need for consensus stems from the lack of a consensus. Why make an issue of agreeing on something that everyone (or nearly everyone) takes for granted? In science, lack of consensus does not bring about the urge to hammer out a consensus by assembling participants whose dogmatic views are well known and who welcome an opportunity to have them reinforced by mutual backslapping.

Naturally, wherever politics holds sway, as night follows day, corruption will abound. An Associated Press article from December 8, 2003, was headlined "Top NIH Officials Paid by Drug Firms." The article began by stating:

> Some of the National Institute of Health's top officials have received hundreds of thousands of dollars in consulting fees from drug companies whose products they were responsible for monitoring, the *Los Angeles Times* reported Sunday.
>
> The newspaper, citing records, reported that in some instances officials of the federal institute operated as consultants for companies whose drugs were linked to the deaths of patients taking part in NIH studies....Medical ethicists said the consulting arrangements are a clear conflict of interest.

The article went on to name two of the senior officials, including "the director of the NIH's Clinical Center, the nation's largest site of medical experiments on humans," and concluded:

> Several other NIH officials were cited as receiving hundreds of thousands of dollars, including one who received more than $1.4 million. Some of them also were paid by companies involved in the agency's research or whose products were the subjects of NIH studies.

## The Commercial Interests

The incentives for the commercial interests are rather obvious. Food manufacturers have been happy to supply low-fat and/or low-cholesterol alternatives—generally at a considerably higher price than the regular fare. Naturally, the companies that have invested heavily in this sort of production are not eager to have people hear that there is no benefit in consuming these "healthy" products.

These companies (usually large conglomerates) also sponsor clinical trials and "studies" to demonstrate the value of their products. No area of the vast food-growing and -production industry is too small or insignificant to try their hands in this. An excellent example came to light a few years back when a study showed that eating walnuts lowered cholesterol levels a bit. This led to a brief boom in walnut consumption. Unfortunately, it soon came out that the "study" was paid for and conducted by a walnut growers association.

The pharmaceutical industry obviously has a huge stake in the survival of the Cholesterol Theory. It is estimated that statin drugs alone bring in $20–$30 billion per year. Add to that the cost of the equipment, chemical reagents, and other paraphernalia for testing not only cholesterol levels but also the liver and muscle enzyme tests required every few weeks, and you get a total expenditure on this one class of drugs that exceeds the gross national product of many countries around the world.

What is not so readily apparent is the degree to which the pharmaceutical companies control the research process itself. They provide the bulk of that portion of the funding that does not come from the taxpayers via the NIH. As mentioned in the last chapter, several of the large trials of statin drugs were designed and executed with the active participation of employees of the companies that manufactured the drugs under investigation. As we saw in the description of just one of the scandals involving NIH personnel, the drug companies are not averse to paying large "consulting" fees to the very people who oversee the testing process.

Because most medical journals are heavily dependent on advertising revenues, which come almost entirely from pharmaceutical firms, it would be naïve to think that editors wouldn't be influenced when selecting articles for publication. Indeed, some people have described the journals of today as little more than marketing arms of the pharmaceutical houses.

## The Medical Profession

The medical profession as a whole and many individual doctors derive great benefit from the anti-cholesterol crusade. The progressive lowering of the "desirable" level of cholesterol has created vast numbers of new "patients" out of the healthy population. According to current guidelines, almost half of the population needs "treatment" for a condition they didn't know they had.

The legitimate duties of a physician consist of helping patients cope with illnesses and medical problems that beset them. This can be a difficult, emotionally stressful, and time-intensive task. Just imagine how a physician would react if someone offered to double or triple his or her volume of patients but with people who are healthy, not complaining of any problems, and taking little of the doctor's precious time. In fact, their interactions would be limited mostly to giving prescriptions and taking blood for testing—tasks that can often be performed by assistants or office staff. It's not that any physicians would deliberately plan such a scenario, but when it's dumped into their laps and they are being told by national authorities that this is the correct thing to do, one can understand why they might not want to invest the time and energy to subject the underlying theory to serious critical review.

The pharmaceutical companies are also willing to go to great lengths to encourage doctors to support the theory and prescribe their products. They flood the physicians' offices with swarms of sales reps or "detail" men and women who help "educate" the doctor about the particular drugs they sell and the diseases those drugs purport to treat. These "detail" people, who, incidentally, include an inordinately large percentage of attractive and vivacious young men and women, come bearing numerous gifts, including drug samples, pens, paperweights, golf equipment, and many other goodies too numerous to list. They also supply meals to the doctors and their office staffs. Some of the local medical offices in my area get a catered lunch virtually every day from different drug houses.

The pharmaceutical companies also sponsor educational conferences for doctors to help them diagnose and treat diseases for which the sponsoring company has drugs to treat. You probably wouldn't be shocked to learn that these meetings are usually held at resorts or other pleasant settings where the participants can also engage in some noneducational pursuits such as gambling, skiing, and golfing, to name a few. Dr. Jerome Kassirer, the former editor of the *New England Journal of Medicine*, has written an entire book on this subject titled *On the Take: How Medicine's Complicity with Big Business Can Endanger Your Health.*

In addition to the material incentives, physicians have a number of non-pecuniary reasons to accept and promulgate the Cholesterol Theory. One is maintenance of credibility. Akin to the researcher who is understandably reluctant to admit that his life's work was essentially worthless is a doctor who has harangued his patients for years about their diet and other personal habits suddenly doing an about-face and admitting that all of that was wrong. Better to accept the "consensus" and not question the premises too closely.

Another motive for physicians is to maintain the fiction of preventive medicine. Many people believe that their doctors play a role in keeping them healthy, and many physicians are not averse to thinking themselves capable of this prodigious task. Unfortunately, the facts speak otherwise. There just isn't really much a doctor can do or recommend to "maintain health" beyond what is commonly known and falls under the heading of motherly advice. For example, cigarette smoking is highly correlated with some (not all) types of lung cancer, and stopping smoking can be a sensible "preventive" measure. But this is certainly known to nearly anyone and doesn't require medical consultation or advice to be known. There is evidence that lowering blood pressure in the truly hypertensive population will reduce the incidence of stroke, but there is not much else.

We know little more about the causes of cancer and how to prevent it than we did 30 years ago. Screening programs for early detection are sold as means of prevention but have had little or no effect on mortality rates. Treatment regimens have provided life extensions measured in weeks or months, but some would say that side effects of the treatment render that extra time moot.

We also know little more about prevention of atherosclerosis (AS) and coronary heat disease (CHD) than we did 30 years ago. Some would say that's because we have been trapped in a blind research alley by the "risk factor" advocates. Many claim that statistics show a gradual decline in CHD mortality over this time. They may even be correct. But if so, it is likely due to improved logistics—the establishment of specialized coronary care units and the advent of paramedic services that provide more rapid transport to the hospital as well as in-the-field defibrillation and CPR—or improved therapeutics such as coronary bypass surgery, anti-platelet drugs, and, more recently, thrombolytic therapy. There is no evidence that "preventive" measures directed at risk-factor modification have had any effect whatsoever.

## The Public

While public acceptance of the diet-heart and cholesterol dogma has no doubt been conditioned by a steady stream of propaganda from the medical authorities and the institutions discussed earlier, there are at least two other elements in the public psyche that have had a profound influence.

One is the normal human desire for control, or, in this case, the illusion of control over one's life and health, and the second is a persistent strain of Puritanical thought that has been part of the American psyche throughout our history.

The best evidence shows that genetics and pure dumb luck are the major determinants of health or disease. But most people don't want to feel like leaves being blown around by the winds of chance. It gives people a certain amount of comfort to feel that they can influence their own fates through proper choices and "clean living." Unfortunately, people's desire for control over the years has repeatedly driven them into the clutches of the charlatans and scam artists. From the snake oil salesmen of the 19th century to the modern purveyors of megavitamins, supplements, and "alternative" therapies such as acupuncture, homeopathy, and chelation, the lure of magic has been irresistible to much of the general public.

As a young physician, I was somewhat taken aback by people's reactions when I explained the facts about cholesterol and diet and their irrelevance to heart disease. Many were upset, and some almost hostile. It took me a while to realize that the resentment came from me threatening the illusion of their control over their health. Patients would often ask me why I didn't believe in the Cholesterol Theory. I would respond that I neither believed nor disbelieved the theory but rather had evidence about the theory. I would try to explain that belief and faith are the province of religion, not science. Some understood, but most preferred the delusion of a "healthy" diet and lifestyle.

The second element that seems ingrained in the human psyche is the feeling that one must suffer to ultimately reap rewards. This belief has its roots in Puritanism, which H.L. Mencken defined as "the haunting fear that someone, somewhere, may be happy." One sees evidence of this in all facets of modern life, but its application to things we eat has a particularly long and rich history. It is no accident that most all of the things we enjoy eating are said to be bad for us. They are given pejorative labels such as "junk food" and "empty calories." Conversely, almost all foods that are bland or distasteful are said to be good for us. Thus, as one author has expressed, "we are supposed to suffer a diet of nutritionally vacuous vegetable matter and inert grain husks (fiber) to gain admittance to the promised land of good health." Applying this sort of Puritanical religiosity to the foods we eat makes no sense either physiologically or nutritionally, but the public accepts it because it appeals to that need for suffering and sacrifice as a prerequisite for achieving the "good."

## Conclusion

We can, from the preceding discussion, begin to get an inkling of why the promoters promote and the medical profession and the public accept an erroneous theory. Two excellent books on the subject are *The Cholesterol Myths* by Uffe Ravnskov and *The Cholesterol Conspiracy* by Russell L. Smith. Both books are well documented, and *The Cholesterol Conspiracy* contains more than 2,500 references. Unfortunately, neither book has achieved the distribution or notoriety they deserve.

Certainly, all the postulates of the Cholesterol Theory fit the definition of myth, and although Dr. Smith makes a persuasive case for conspiracy, that may be an unfortunate choice of words because most of the public has been persuaded to dismiss out of hand anyone who proposes such things as "just a conspiracy theorist." Surely there has been conspiracy as Dr. Smith defines it, which is simply two or more people or groups working together for common ends. Thus, conspiracy may be for either good or evil purposes, but we have seen from the preceding discussion that it is not necessary to claim conspiracy when it comes to cholesterol. One can see how the theory evolved by groups independently pursuing their self-interests and responding to the incentives before them. The acceptance of the theory by the medical profession and the public may be understood in much the same way. Therefore, I feel the proper term is "delusion" as defined in the beginning of this book. The delusion persists because it serves some purposes and fills some needs.

The historian Daniel J. Boorstin once wrote, "The greatest obstacle to discovery is not ignorance—it is the illusion of knowledge." When I was a youngster, we were told that eating "greasy" foods, chocolate, or anything else that teenagers like to eat would cause outbreaks of acne. There was nothing that we hated or feared more than that. Of course there was never any scientific evidence behind this concept and it has now been discarded. But it took many years to rid ourselves of what we "knew" to be true about foods and acne. Hopefully, the Cholesterol Theory will also end up in the ash heap of discredited ideas, but only time will tell.

# AFTERWORD

I stated at the outset of this book that it is logically impossible to prove a nega-tive construct. Rather, the burden of proof is always on the person making a pos-itive statement about cause and effect in scientific phenomena. All we can do is examine the evidence given by a proponent of any particular theory and see if it stands up to scientific scrutiny.

We have seen that the proponents of the Cholesterol and Diet-Heart Theories have failed this test. But if these theories are to be discarded, what will take their place?

This is a question to which there is no certain answer at this time. But we might be able to make some intelligent guesses about where to look by going back to fundamentals and looking at what we *do* know about the pathology of athero-sclerosis (AS) and coronary heart disease (CHD).

To do this, let's revisit some of the basics of AS that were listed at the end of Chapter 3:

—-Atherosclerosis primarily affects the arteries—those blood vessels that carry blood under relatively high pressures. The veins carry the blood under low pres-sure (1/20 to 1/100 that of the arteries) and almost never show evidence of AS, but when the veins are subjected to arterial pressures by being used for coronary bypass grafts or as part of an arteriovenous fistula for dialysis patients, they show the rapid development of AS.

—-Atherosclerosis doesn't affect all portions of a given artery. There is a marked tendency for AS to develop at branching points and along the lesser curvatures, where the physical stress on the wall of the artery is the greatest. It is very commonly seen that one side of the arterial wall is severely atherosclerotic while the opposite side is virtually normal.

—-Atherosclerosis is ubiquitous. It is found in all people and all animals, including those that are strict vegetarians. The earliest changes are detectable in newborn infants, and the degree of AS progresses steadily with age.

All of these factors suggest that hemodynamic stress on the wall of the blood vessel is a more likely causative factor for AS than some chemical circulating in the blood. Is AS a "normal" protective response designed to allow the arterial wall to better withstand the stresses caused by high pressure blood flow? Does the thickening and rigidification of the arterial wall provide this protection? Perhaps.

Why do some people develop a more severe form of AS and at an earlier age than most? What is it about the diabetes that seems to accelerate this process? Why do some people suffer heart attacks and strokes while others with the same degree of AS do not? Why does the occurrence of heart attacks at relatively young ages seem to run in families?

These are all excellent questions. Unfortunately, the "risk factor" paradigm for investigating the causes of degenerative diseases such as AS has provided no answers. Nor is it likely to do so. To advance our understanding of AS and start to get some answers to these seminal questions, we must break out of the risk-factor paradigm in which AS research has been trapped for decades.

In his classic book, *The Structure of Scientific Revolutions*, Thomas S. Kuhn showed that science doesn't really advance much by successive small steps but rather through dramatic shifts in the general paradigm that scientists use as a framework for their theories of causation. A paradigm is a philosophical or theoretical framework or way of looking at certain phenomena in the real world. Kuhn points out that a paradigm based on faulty assumptions will be faced with steadily increasing amounts of contradictory data. The facts that don't fit the existing paradigm will at first be rationalized but will eventually so complicate the theoretical framework that the entire paradigm must shift and incorporate new assumptions that will better explain the facts that contradicted the old framework or paradigm.

A classic example of this sort of paradigm shift is in the field of astronomy. The ancient system described by Ptolemy placed the earth at the center of the universe with the sun and other planets rotating around it. This was known as the geocentric system. Using this system, the ancients could roughly predict the motion of the planets. But as new data became available that contradicted the expectations of the existing model, they had to make adjustments to make the new facts fit the existing theory. Initially, they postulated small epicycles superimposed on the larger planetary orbits to explain the contradictory data, but as the epicycles multiplied, they caused the entire system to become so hopelessly complex that it had to be discarded. Fortunately, Copernicus came along and proposed a system with the sun at the center and the earth and the other planets rotating about it. This is known as the heliocentric system, and, with this new paradigm, the predictions of planetary motion became much simpler and more accurate.

One can look at the paradigm for the causation of AS in much the same way. The early theorists placed cholesterol at the center of the system and built their theories around it. As contradictory data came to light, modifications were made to explain away the contradictions. For example, when it was shown that there were lots of people with high cholesterol and no disease as well as those with severe disease but normal or low cholesterol levels, it was postulated that there is both "good" and "bad" cholesterol (HDL and LDL). When it was shown that LDL ("bad" cholesterol) didn't really correlate well with AS and its complications, it was said that "oxidized" LDL was the culprit.

And so it goes.

Until we realize that the basic assumption that cholesterol is the central key is wrong, there will likely be little progress in answering the important questions. The whole point of this book is to show that cholesterol is not only not the *central* factor but no factor at all.

# How to Read a Medical Journal Report

Medical journal reports usually follow a prescribed pattern. Below the title and list of authors is an abstract or summary written by the authors. There then follows an introductory section where background information is given on the problem to be investigated. This introduction is designed to provide context for the report. The next section is usually titled "Methods" or sometimes "Patients and Methods." Here, the authors describe the nuts and bolts of the study: how it was designed, how the subjects were selected, what the end points are, how the statistical analysis is to be done, and so on. Next comes a section titled "Results"; this is really the guts of the paper, where the authors report the numbers. The final section of the paper is usually titled "Discussion" or "Conclusion." Here the authors give their impression of what the study showed and speculate on the implications for treatment, further research, etc.

The easiest way to analyze a study is to break it down into these sections and discuss what to look for under each heading.

1)  Summary or Abstract: Read this to get an overview of what is to come, but don't take it too seriously, as it often reflects the subjective impressions of the authors.

2) Introduction: Approach this the same was as the Summary or Abstract. The authors will often include matter-of-fact statements about conclusions or theories that are highly debatable. These are often self-serving and should be taken with a grain of salt.

3) Methods: This section is crucial. How were the patients selected and who was excluded? What are the sources for the data, and how were they collected? How reliable are they? Ask yourself whether the end points are hard or soft. Total mortality is always a hard end point. All others are up for grabs. How is cause of death determined? If death certificates or verbal reports from family members or the patient's physician are used, be very skeptical of any statistics related to cause of death. Remember that symptom-related end points (for example, chest pain or exercise tolerance) are very subjective and, therefore, relatively worthless. Ask whether the study is double-blinded so that neither the subjects nor the investigators can tell who is getting the real drug or treatment versus the placebo. If not, then bias can creep in and invalidate the results.

4) Results: As mentioned earlier, this section is the guts of the study. Most papers will print a table that summarizes the results of each end point for each experimental group. They should list the raw numbers and the calculated percentage of the total group (absolute risk). Those are the only figures that matter. Authors will often also list relative risk-reduction figures, but these can be ignored. Any report that gives only the relative risk figures and omits the raw data and/or absolute risk figures is likely

engaging in deception, so any conclusions it draws should be viewed with great skepticism.

Authors will almost always list a "p "value for each end point. P values are supposed to tell you whether a difference found between two groups is statistically significant. You should ignore these and simply compare the differences in absolute risk and use common sense to tell you if the differences are of any practical significance.

For example, say you are testing a drug and have 1,000 patients each in the treatment and control groups. During the trial, 2 patients in the treatment group and 4 in the control group die. The absolute risks are 0.2% and 0.4% respectively. The absolute risk reduction is 0.2%, but the relative risk reduction is 50%, which sounds a lot more impressive. The p value may indicate that the tiny difference between the two groups is statistically significant, but this is irrelevant, because common sense tells you that the difference is of no practical significance.

Any study that doesn't give the actual numbers for the raw data and absolute risk can be dismissed out of hand. Some reports will give the raw data in tabular form but never mention it in the text of the article. Rather, the authors will present a variety of derivative statistical measures such as risk ratios and complicated regression formulas. Ignore all of these and seek out the basic numbers. Assume that if the basic numbers are not given, the authors are hiding something.

5) Discussion: In this section, the authors analyze the significance of their findings. How do their conclusions match up with your analysis of the key numbers in the raw data? Do they use hyperbole when it is not warranted by the data, for example, describing correlations as strong that are obviously not? If so, you can be sure the authors are engaging in advocacy and not science. Do they extrapolate their results to apply to populations beyond that justified by the data? Do they make grandiose claims about the significance of their conclusions? These are all indicators of possible bias on the part of the authors and should cast a cloud of suspicion over the entire report.

6) The Fine Print: Examine this carefully. It is usually located at the bottom left of the first page and/or at the end of the report. The fine print lists the institutions that participated in the study and, more importantly, who financed the study. Although science should be objective and "value-free," the truth is that most institutions, like individuals, have their own agendas and pet theories. For example, it's probably safe to bet that one can't find a single study critical of the Cholesterol Theory that was sponsored or financed by the American Heart Institute (AHA) or National Heart, Lung, and Blood Institute (NHLBI). If a drug study is financed, planned, or monitored by the company manufacturing the drug under investigation, be very skeptical about the honesty of the report.

Examples of the application of the method of analysis I have described in this appendix are given for the two studies most commonly cited as "proving" the Cholesterol Theory. Appendix II contains the original article on the Lipid Research Clinics Trial followed by a detailed critical analysis. Appendix III does the same with the Helsinki Heart Study.

# APPENDIX II

A. Original Report of the Lipid Research Clinics Trial

B. How to Read and Interpret the LRC-CPPT Report

## Original Contributions

# The Lipid Research Clinics Coronary Primary Prevention Trial Results

## I. Reduction in Incidence of Coronary Heart Disease

Lipid Research Clinics Program

● The Lipid Research Clinics Coronary Primary Prevention Trial (LRC-CPPT), a multicenter, randomized, double-blind study, tested the efficacy of cholesterol lowering in reducing risk of coronary heart disease (CHD) in 3,806 asymptomatic middle-aged men with primary hypercholesterolemia (type II hyperlipoproteinemia). The treatment group received the bile acid sequestrant cholestyramine resin and the control group received a placebo for an average of 7.4 years. Both groups followed a moderate cholesterol-lowering diet. The cholestyramine group experienced average plasma total and low-density lipoprotein cholesterol (LDL-C) reductions of 13.4% and 20.3%, respectively, which were 8.5% and 12.6% greater reductions than those obtained in the placebo group. The cholestyramine group experienced a 19% reduction in risk ($P<.05$) of the primary end point—definite CHD death and/or definite nonfatal myocardial infarction—reflecting a 24% reduction in definite CHD death and a 19% reduction in nonfatal myocardial infarction. The cumulative seven-year incidence of the primary end point was 7% in the cholestyramine group v 8.6% in the placebo group. In addition, the incidence rates for new positive exercise tests, angina, and coronary bypass surgery were reduced by 25%, 20%, and 21%, respectively, in the cholestyramine group. The risk of death from all causes was only slightly and not significantly reduced in the cholestyramine group. The magnitude of this decrease (7%) was less than for CHD end points because of a greater number of violent and accidental deaths in the cholestyramine group. The LRC-CPPT findings show that reducing total cholesterol by lowering LDL-C levels can diminish the incidence of CHD morbidity and mortality in men at high risk for CHD because of raised LDL-C levels. This clinical trial provides strong evidence for a causal role for these lipids in the pathogenesis of CHD.

(JAMA 1984;251:351-364)

CORONARY heart disease (CHD) remains the major cause of death and disability in the United States and in other industrialized countries despite recent declines in CHD mortality rates. It accounts for more deaths annually than any other disease, including all forms of cancer combined.[1] Nationally, more than 1 million heart attacks occur each year and more than a half million people still die as a result. Coronary heart disease ranks first in terms of social security disability, second only to all forms of arthritis for limitation of activity and all forms of cancer combined for total hospital bed days. In direct health care costs, lost wages, and productivity, CHD costs the United States more than $60 billion a year.

This enormous toll has focused attention on the possible prevention of CHD by various means, especially through lowering of the plasma cholesterol level. Observational epidemiologic studies have established that the higher the plasma total or low-density lipoprotein cholesterol (LDL-C) level, the greater the risk that CHD will develop.[2] The view that LDL-C is intimately involved in atherogenesis, the basic pathophysiologic process responsible for most CHD, is sustained by reports from other epidemiologic studies as well as many animal experiments, pathological observations, clinical investigations, and metabolic ward studies.[3]

Plasma total and LDL-C levels may be reduced by diets and drugs. However, before such treatment can be advocated with confidence and before it can be concluded that cholesterol plays a causal role in the pathogenesis of CHD, it is desirable to show that reducing cholesterol levels safely reduces the risk of CHD in man. Many clinical trials of cholesterol lowering have been conducted, but their results, although often encouraging, have been inconclusive.

The most appropriate clinical trial of the efficacy of cholesterol lowering would be a dietary study, because of the links between diets high in saturated fat and cholesterol typical of most industrialized populations, high plasma total and LDL-C levels, and a

From the Lipid Metabolism-Atherogenesis Branch, National Heart, Lung, and Blood Institute, Bethesda, Md.

Reprint requests to Lipid Metabolism-Atherogenesis Branch, National Heart, Lung, and Blood Institute, Federal 401, Bethesda, MD 20205 (Basil M. Rifkind, MD).

high incidence of CHD. However, the 1971 National Heart and Lung Institute Task Force on Arteriosclerosis recommended against conducting a large-scale, national diet-heart trial in the general population because of concern regarding the blinding of such a study, the large sample size, and the prohibitive cost, then estimated to range from $500 million to more than $1 billion.[4] Accordingly, the Lipid Research Clinics Coronary Primary Prevention Trial (LRC-CPPT) was initiated in 1973 as an alternative test of the efficacy of reducing cholesterol levels. The choice of hypercholesterolemic men at high risk of CHD events developing reduced the necessary sample size to a feasible level; in this regard, women were not recruited because of their lower risk of CHD.

The use of the drug cholestyramine resin permitted a double-blind design. This drug, previously approved for general use by the Food and Drug Administration, was selected on account of its known effectiveness in reducing total cholesterol and LDL-C levels,[5] the availability of a suitable placebo, its nonabsorbability from the gastrointestinal (GI) tract, its few systemic effects, and its low level of significant toxicity.

Reported herein is the outcome of the study with respect to its major response variables, definite CHD death and/or definite nonfatal myocardial infarction, and related data.

## PARTICIPANTS AND METHODS

The design of the LRC-CPPT has been described in detail.[4] Briefly, the LRC-CPPT was a double-blind, placebo-controlled clinical trial that tested the efficacy of lowering cholesterol levels for primary prevention of CHD. Twelve participating Lipid Research Clinics (LRCs) recruited 3,806 middle-aged men with primary hypercholesterolemia (type II hyperlipoproteinemia) free of, but at high risk for, CHD because of elevated LDL-C levels. The men were randomized into two groups that were similar in baseline characteristics. The treatment group received the bile acid sequestrant cholestyramine resin, and the control group received a placebo; both groups followed a moderate cholesterol-lowering diet. To ensure comparability of all data across the 12 clinics over a ten-year period, a common protocol documenting all procedures in detail was strictly adhered to by clinical personnel, who were trained and certified in stan-

dardized procedures.[7] All aspects of the conduct of the study were carefully monitored by the Central Patient Registry and Coordinating Center and by the Program Office. The progress of the trial and the possibility of serious side effects were reviewed twice a year by a Safety and Data Monitoring Board. Any protocol violations that were identified were brought to the attention of this board; none were regarded by them to put the trial into jeopardy.

### Selection of Participants

The LRCs recruited men aged 35 to 59 years with a plasma cholesterol level of 265 mg/dL or greater (the 95th percentile for 1,364 men aged 40 to 49 years who participated in a previous LRC pilot study) and with an LDL-C level of 190 mg/dL or greater. Men with triglyceride levels averaging greater than 300 mg/dL or with type III hyperlipoproteinemia were excluded.

The numerous sources of the volunteer participants and the techniques of their recruitment have been described.[8,9] Of the approximately 480,000 age-eligible men screened between July 1973 and July 1976, 3,810 were eventually entered into the trial.[10] Four, two in each treatment group, were subsequently removed when they were found to have type III hyperlipoproteinemia, and the results reported are for the 3,806 type II participants. The participants were preponderantly college- or high school-educated whites. Their mean age was 47.8 years. Informed consent was obtained from each participant randomized into the study.

Participants were also excluded if they had any of the following clinical manifestations of CHD: (1) history of definite or suspect myocardial infarction; (2) angina pectoris, as determined by Rose Questionnaire; (3) angina pectoris during exercise electrocardiography; (4) various ECG abnormalities, according to the Minnesota code—left bundle-branch block, tertiary or secondary heart block, two or more consecutive ventricular premature beats, left ventricular hypertrophy, R-on-T-type ventricular premature beats, or atrial flutter or fibrillation; or (5) congestive heart failure. Men with a positive exercise test result in the absence of other manifestations of CHD were not excluded. Only men in good health and free of conditions associated with secondary hyperlipoproteinemia, such as diabetes mellitus, hypothyroidism, nephrotic syndrome, hepatic disease, hyperuricemia, and notable obesity, were selected. Men were excluded if they had hypertension or were receiving antihypertensive medication or had life-limiting or comorbid conditions such as cancer or nonatherosclerotic cardiovascular disease. Men who required long-term

use of certain other medications were also excluded.

### Screening (Prerandomization) Visits

The accrual phase consisted of four screening visits at monthly intervals. Physical examinations, lipid and lipoprotein level determinations, clinical chemistry measurements, medical history ascertainment, and resting and graded exercise ECGs were performed. At the second screening visit, a moderate cholesterol-lowering diet, which aimed to provide 400 mg of cholesterol per day and a polyunsaturated-to-saturated fat ratio of approximately 0.8 and which was designed to lower cholesterol levels 3% to 5%, was prescribed for all potential participants.[4]

A cholesterol-lowering diet was offered to potential participants because, when the LRC-CPPT began, it was the practice of many physicians to recommend such a diet to hypercholesterolemic patients. Although the cholesterol lowering expected from the diet given to both study groups had the potential to diminish the statistical power of the trial by reducing the subsequent incidence of CHD, it was hoped that such a diet, along with a nutritional counseling program, would facilitate recruitment of participants. Moreover, since the diet was introduced before randomization, it was possible to exclude men whose plasma cholesterol levels were highly sensitive to diet. Thus, men whose LDL-C levels fell below 175 mg/dL at the third or fourth screening visit were excluded. The maintenance of both treatment groups on the diet after randomization minimized the opportunity for confounding of the study because of differential dietary intakes. Dietary intake was assessed semiannually by means of a 24-hour dietary recall.[11]

### Randomization

At the fifth visit to the clinic, eligible participants were randomly divided by the permuted block method into two treatment groups within eight prognostic strata at each of the 12 clinics. The strata were based on high and low risk of CHD with respect to LDL-C level ($\geq$ or <215 mg/dL), ST-segment depression during exercise testing, and a logistic risk function of age, cigarette smoking, and diastolic blood pressure.

Only five of 83 variables compared at baseline showed statistically significant differences (height, weight, and two-hour postchallenge glucose, SGOT, and albumin levels).[10] Because the observed differences were small and the number of statistically significant differences is that expected by chance in comparisons involving a large number of variables, the randomization and stratification process was found to produce two almost identical groups.

## Study Medication

Participants were prescribed either the bile acid sequestrant cholestyramine resin at 24 g/day (six packets per day, divided into two to four equal doses) or an equivalent amount of placebo, dispensed in identical sealed packets. Those unable to tolerate six packets per day were prescribed a reduced dosage. Rigorous steps such as unique marking of individual packets and boxes and continuous external auditing of medications were followed to ensure proper drug-allocation assignment. Medication adherence was monitored by means of a packet count (packets issued minus packets returned, divided by the number of days elapsed since the packets were issued).

## Postrandomization Visits

Participants attended clinics every two months, at which time the study medication was dispensed, dietary and drug counseling was given, and end points and possible drug side effects, as well as possible confounding variables such as blood pressure and weight, were evaluated. Intervention by LRC-CPPT staff was restricted to prescription of the study medication and the diet. At annual and/or semiannual visits, resting and graded exercise ECGs, 24-hour dietary recalls, and complete physical examinations and medical histories were obtained. All participants initially entered were followed up to the completion of the trial irrespective of their levels of adherence and the frequency of their visits.

## Lipid Measurements

Lipid levels were determined with high precision and accuracy. Comparability of the measurements of the 12 LRC laboratories was ensured by a rigorous quality control program especially designed for the LRC Program and maintained by the Lipid Standardization Laboratory. The lipid levels at the second screening (prediet) visit were used as the baseline to calculate the changes in levels of total cholesterol and LDL-C and triglyceride observed at subsequent visits. Since the measurement of HDL-cholesterol (HDL-C) levels at the second screening visit was not performed according to protocol at several clinics, the levels at the first screening visit were used as the baseline to calculate change in HDL-C levels.

## End Points

The primary end point for evaluating the treatment was the combination of definite CHD death and/or definite nonfatal myocardial infarction. Appendix A gives the detailed definitions of these events as well as the definition of suspect CHD death and suspect nonfatal myocar-

dial infarction. Other end points included all-cause mortality, the development of an ischemic ECG response to exercise (positive exercise test result), angina pectoris as determined by Rose Questionnaire, atherothrombotic brain infarction, arterial peripheral vascular disease (intermittent claudication as determined by Rose Questionnaire), and transient cerebral ischemic attack. Detailed definitions of these nonprimary end points have been published elsewhere.[5]

The classification of cause of death was based on the examination of death certificates, hospital records, and interviews with physicians, witnesses of the death, and next of kin. The diagnosis of nonfatal myocardial infarction was based on ECGs, blood enzyme levels, and history of chest pain at the time of the clinical event. A physician at the clinic at which the potential end point occurred classified the end point. In addition, each potential end point was classified independently by two members of a blinded verification panel. If the three reviewers agreed, the diagnosis was accepted. If there was disagreement, the case was submitted for definitive classification to the LRC-CPPT Cardiovascular Endpoints Committee.[5] Classification of deaths not caused by CHD was also performed by a blinded panel.

An intraoperative event was classified on the basis of ECG changes occurring during coronary bypass surgery or other cardiac surgery or during the recovery period extending from the time of surgery until discharge from the hospital.

## Statistical Methods

The hypothesis of the LRC-CPPT was that lowering cholesterol (or LDL-C) levels would reduce the incidence of end points, and, hence, a one-sided test was used for the main hypothesis. The statistic reported is a stratified (using the eight baseline risk strata) log rank (Mantel-Haenszel) statistic.[12] This statistic compares the life-table survival (or failure) curves in the two groups rather than the proportion of failures. In view of the necessity for periodic review, the data were analyzed many times, and conventional methods of computing statistical significance no longer applied. Several statistical methods were used to monitor the trial. These methods included a modification of the method of O'Brien and Fleming,[13] the two-dimensional rank statistic of Majundar and Sen,[14] and a modification of the method of Breslow and Haug.[15] All of these methods essentially gave the same result, and, in view of its ease of presentation, the modified O'Brien and Fleming method was used for this article. As formulated by O'Brien and Fleming, the data are analyzed $k$ times after an equal number of end points. In

practice, the data for this trial were analyzed at 15 equal time intervals, and strictly speaking, the method of determining the critical value proposed by O'Brien and Fleming does not hold. The distribution of the statistic taking into account the actual times when the analyses were conducted was determined by simulation and the critical $z$ value for a one-sided test with $\alpha=0.05$ was found to be 1.87, as compared with the O'Brien-Fleming value of 1.83. The simulated critical value 1.87 is used in this report.

This method for determining significance was used for the primary end point of the study. Other statistical tests reported use the nominal level of significance. The reader is cautioned that interpretation of these nominal $P$ values should include the possibility that some may be significant by chance because of the many comparisons made.

The Kaplan-Meier method was used for construction of the life-table plots.[12] The percentage reduction of end points is reported as $(1-RR)\times100$, where $RR$ is the estimated relative risk of an event in the cholestyramine group, compared with the placebo group. For end points where time of occurrence could be obtained precisely, the relative risk was estimated from the life tables. Where the actual time of occurrence (eg, the onset of angina) could not be precisely determined, the relative risk was estimated from the 2×2 table defined by treatment and the occurrence of an end point. All relative risks were estimated, taking into account the baseline risk strata, unless otherwise noted.

To conform with the one-sided test of the main hypothesis, 90% confidence intervals for the estimated reduction in risk are reported. The Cox proportional hazards model[12] was used to adjust the treatment comparisons for other variables, such as blood pressure. Tests of interaction in the proportional hazards model were accomplished by including cross-product terms in the model.

Homogeneity of treatment effect over risk strata was assessed by an efficient scores test based on the proportional hazards model and included parameters for treatment and strata.[14] Homogeneity of effect over clinic was similarly assessed.

## RESULTS

### Follow-up

All men were followed up for a minimum of seven and up to ten years. The average period of follow-up was 7.4 years. Between May 15 and Aug 27, 1983, contact was made with all of the men who were still living, including any who discontinued visits during the course of the trial. Thus, the vital status is known for all men

| Table 1.—Median Daily Dietary Intake | | | | | | | | |
|---|---|---|---|---|---|---|---|---|
| | Placebo | | | | Cholestyramine Resin | | | |
| | Pre-entry | | Postentry | | Pre-entry | | Postentry | |
| Dietary Variable | Prediet | On-Diet | 1st Year | 7th Year | Prediet | On-Diet | 1st Year | 7th Year |
| Total calories | 2,264 | 2,023 | 2,056 | 2,060 | 2,278 | 2,027 | 2,058 | 2,066 |
| Cholesterol, mg | 309 | 248 | 255 | 284 | 308 | 243 | 251 | 266 |
| Total fat, g | 95 | 79 | 83 | 87 | 97 | 80 | 82 | 89 |
| Saturated fat, g | 33 | 24 | 26 | 28 | 34 | 24 | 26 | 29 |
| P/S* ratio | 0.48 | 0.73 | 0.69 | 0.67 | 0.47 | 0.72 | 0.67 | 0.66 |

*Ratio of polyunsaturated fats to saturated fats.

| Table 2.—Mean Plasma Lipid and Lipoprotein Cholesterol Concentrations | | | | | | | | |
|---|---|---|---|---|---|---|---|---|
| | Placebo | | | | Cholestyramine Resin | | | |
| | Pre-entry | | Postentry | | Pre-entry | | Postentry | |
| Lipid | Prediet | On-Diet | 1st Year | 7th Year | Prediet | On-Diet | 1st Year | 7th Year |
| Total cholesterol, mg/dL | 291.8 | 279.2 | 275.4 | 277.3 | 291.5 | 280.4 | 238.6 | 257.1 |
| LDL* cholesterol, mg/dL | 216.2 | 204.5 | 198.8 | 197.6 | 215.6 | 205.3 | 159.4 | 174.9 |
| HDL* cholesterol, mg/dL | 45.1 | 44.4 | 44.5 | 45.5 | 45.0 | 44.4 | 45.6 | 46.6 |
| HDL cholesterol/total cholesterol | 0.16 | 0.16 | 0.16 | 0.17 | 0.16 | 0.16 | 0.20 | 0.19 |
| Triglycerides, mg/dL | 158.4 | 153.2 | 162.0 | 173.5 | 159.8 | 156.3 | 172.2 | 182.9 |

*LDL indicates low-density lipoprotein; HDL, high-density lipoprotein.

originally entered into the study. In addition, every man or a close relative was questioned before and at the end of the study regarding previous hospitalizations for CHD or other reasons.

### Adherence to Treatment

During the first year, the mean daily packet count for participants attending clinic was 4.2 in the cholestyramine and 4.9 in the placebo group, falling to 3.8 and 4.6, respectively, by the seventh year. Adherence to the diet as determined by a 24-hour dietary recall conducted at six-month intervals showed no important differences between the two treatment groups (Table 1). A rise of 2 kg in body weight occurred in each group during the seven years of the study.

### Maintenance of Blind

No cases of medical emergency required the unblinding of participants or staff and no one asked to be told his treatment assignment.

### Lipids and Lipoproteins

When the LRC-CPPT diet was introduced, total cholesterol levels fell $11.1 \pm 0.65$ (mean $\pm$ SE) mg/dL in the cholestyramine group and $12.6 \pm 0.67$ mg/dL in the placebo group

(Table 2). Corresponding falls of $10.3 \pm 0.61$ and $11.7 \pm 0.63$ mg/dL occurred in LDL-C levels. During the first year of follow-up, there were additional falls of $41.8 \pm 0.81$ mg/dL and $45.9 \pm 0.82$ mg/dL in total and LDL-C levels in the cholestyramine group and $3.8 \pm 0.51$ mg/dL and $5.7 \pm 0.48$ mg/dL in the placebo group. By seven years, the total and LDL-C levels had fallen, from the pre-entry postdiet levels, $23.3 \pm 0.99$ mg/dL and $30.4 \pm 0.99$ mg/dL in the cholestyramine group and $1.9 \pm 0.75$ mg/dL and $6.9 \pm 0.70$ mg/dL in the placebo group. Almost all of the change in total cholesterol was in the LDL-C fraction. During treatment, the cholestyramine group experienced average plasma total cholesterol and LDL-C reductions of 13.4% and 20.3%, respectively, which were 8.5% and 12.6% greater ($P<.001$) than those obtained in the placebo group. (It should be noted that these percentage changes were computed for each individual and then averaged.) There was a $1.6 \pm 0.19$-mg/dL increase in HDL-C levels and a larger increase in triglyceride levels attributable to cholestyramine therapy. There also was a rise in triglyceride levels in the placebo group, although not as great as in the cholestyramine group. Additional details are provided in the companion article.[17]

### Primary End Point

The cholestyramine group experienced 155 definite CHD deaths and/or definite nonfatal myocardial infarctions, whereas the placebo group had 187 such events (Table 3). When the stratified log rank test was used to take into account the stratification of participants at entry and their differing lengths of follow-up, the incidence rate of CHD was estimated to be 19% lower in the cholestyramine than in the placebo group. The $z$ score for this difference was 1.92 with $P<.05$, after adjustment for multiple looks at the data. Both the fatal and nonfatal categories of the primary end points showed corresponding reductions. Thirty CHD deaths occurred in the cholestyramine group as compared with 38 CHD deaths in the placebo group, representing a reduction in risk of 24%. The cholestyramine group experienced 130 definite nonfatal myocardial infarctions, compared with 158 in the placebo group, with a 19% reduction in risk. The inclusion of the categories of suspect CHD death and suspect nonfatal myocardial infarction resulted in an overall reduction in risk of 15%, with a 30% reduction for fatal events and a 15% reduction for nonfatal events. The $z$ score for this comparison exceeded the nominal 5% threshold (1.65) for statistical significance and

| Table 3.—Definite or Suspect Primary End Points and All-Cause Mortality | | | | | | | | |
|---|---|---|---|---|---|---|---|---|
| | Placebo (N=1,900) | | Cholestyramine Resin (N=1,906) | | % Reduction in Risk* | 90% Confidence Interval for % Reduction in Risk | | z Score |
| End Point | No. | % | No. | % | | | | |
| Definite coronary heart disease (CHD) death and/or definite nonfatal myocardial infarction | 187† | 9.8 | 155† | 8.1 | 19 | +3 | +32 | 1.92‡ |
| Definite CHD death | 38 | 2.0 | 30 | 1.6 | 24 | ... | ... | ... |
| Definite nonfatal myocardial infarction | 158 | 8.3 | 130 | 6.8 | 19 | ... | ... | ... |
| Definite or suspect CHD death or nonfatal myocardial infarction | 256† | 13.5 | 222† | 11.6 | 15 | +1 | +27 | 1.80 |
| Definite or suspect CHD death | 44 | 2.3 | 32 | 1.7 | 30 | ... | ... | ... |
| Definite or suspect nonfatal myocardial infarction | 225 | 11.8 | 195 | 10.2 | 15 | ... | ... | ... |
| All-cause mortality | 71 | 3.7 | 68 | 3.6 | 7 | −23 | +30 | 0.42 |

*Percent reduction in risk is defined as $(1-RR) \times 100\%$, where $RR$ is the incidence rate ratio of an event in the cholestyramine group compared with the placebo. Percent reduction in risk and z score are adjusted for follow-up time and stratification.
†A subject experiencing a myocardial infarction and CHD death is counted once in this category. Hence, this line is not the sum of the following two lines.
‡The .05-level, one-sided critical value of the z score adjusted for multiple looks at the data is 1.87.

was close to the modified O'Brien-Fleming threshold of 1.87 (see "Participants and Methods" section). Thus, the conclusion that treatment was beneficial is not essentially altered by the inclusion of suspect events. The separate category of intraoperative myocardial infarction (Table 4) also showed more cases in the placebo group (7 v 5), although the difference is not statistically significant. (One of the four type III participants excluded after the randomization experienced a nonfatal myocardial infarction; he was in the placebo group.)

The life-table failure rates in the two groups are plotted in the Figure. Very early in the follow-up period, the number of CHD events was higher in the cholestyramine group, but by two years the two curves were identical. Thereafter, there was a steady divergence of the two sets of event rates, and at seven years of follow-up the event rate was 8.6% in the placebo group and 7.0% in the cholestyramine group, a reduction of 19%.

The primary end points were examined within the risk strata defined at randomization. The hypothesis of homogeneity of effect across these strata was not rejected. Thus, although differences were observed in the estimated relative risk among the strata, there was insufficient statistical evidence to claim that the treatment was more beneficial in one stratum than in another. The cholestyramine-treated group at seven clinics had at least 18% fewer primary

| Table 4.—Other Cardiovascular Events* | | | | | |
|---|---|---|---|---|---|
| | Placebo (N=1,900) | | Cholestyramine Resin (N=1,906) | | % Reduction in Risk |
| End Point | No. | % | No. | % | |
| Coronary disease | | | | | |
| Positive exercise test | 345 | 19.8† | 260 | 14.9† | 25‡ |
| Angina (Rose Questionnaire) | 287 | 15.1† | 235 | 12.4† | 20‡ |
| Coronary bypass surgery | 112 | 5.9 | 93 | 4.9 | 21‡ |
| Congestive heart failure | 11 | 0.6 | 8 | 0.4 | 28 |
| Intraoperative myocardial infarction | 7 | 0.4 | 5 | 0.3 | 29 |
| Resuscitated coronary collapse | 5 | 0.3 | 3 | 0.2 | 40 |
| Cerebrovascular disease | | | | | |
| Definite or suspect transient cerebral ischemic attack | 22 | 1.2 | 18 | 0.9 | 18 |
| Definite or suspect atherothrombotic brain infarction | 14 | 0.7 | 17 | 0.9 | −21 |
| Peripheral vascular disease | | | | | |
| Intermittent claudication (Rose Questionnaire) | 84 | 4.4† | 72 | 3.8† | 15‡ |

*Counts all events for each individual, including events occurring after a nonfatal myocardial infarction.
†Percent of those without condition at baseline.
‡Percent reduction in risk is adjusted for stratification.

end points than placebo-treated men. At four clinics there was essentially no treatment difference; only one clinic showed an excess of events in the drug group. The statistical hypothesis of homogeneity of effect among clinics also was not rejected; thus, the benefit of cholestyramine resin treatment cannot be attributed to effects in only a small number of clinics.

This stratified analysis provided an estimate of treatment benefit adjusted for baseline strata of what were considered to be the most important CHD risk factors when the study began. Adjustment for a more extensive list of baseline characteristics, including LDL-C, HDL-C, triglycer-

ide, age, cigarette smoking, and systolic blood pressure, each considered as a continuous variable, as well as exercise test outcome, was performed by Cox proportional hazards analysis. The adjusted estimates of treatment effect (20.0% risk reduction) and z score (2.05) were slightly greater than those obtained in the stratified analysis. There was no significant interaction of the treatment effect with any of the seven baseline characteristics. Thus, the proportional hazards and stratified analyses both indicate that it is highly unlikely that the treatment benefit could have arisen from inequality of the two treatment groups with respect to CHD risk at baseline or from a par-

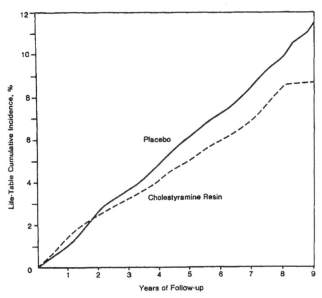

N=3,806   3,753   3,701   3,659   3,615   3,564   3,520   3,466   1,816   302

Life-table cumulative incidence of primary end point (definite coronary heart disease death and / or definite nonfatal myocardial infarction) in treatment groups, computed by Kaplan-Meier method. N equals total number of Lipid Research Clinics Coronary Primary Prevention Trial participants at risk for their first primary end point, followed at each time point.

ticular subgroup of LRC-CPPT participants.

### Other Cardiovascular End Points

The frequency of other cardiovascular end points in the two treatment groups is reported in Table 4. Each of the CHD categories having a large number of events showed a reduction in incidence similar to the 19% reduction in the primary end point. Thus, the cholestyramine group showed reductions of 20% (P<.01) in the incidence of the development of angina ascertained by the Rose Questionnaire, 25% (P<.001) in the development of a new positive exercise test result, and 21% (P=.06) in incidence of coronary bypass surgery. The two cerebrovascular disease categories did not provide a consistent or significant pattern of benefit, but the numbers were small. For peripheral vascular disease there was a 15% (P>.1) reduction in new intermittent claudication in the cholestyramine group. None of the other differences in Table 4 were statistically significant, possibly because of the small numbers.

### All-Cause Mortality

Although the incidence of definite and of definite and suspect CHD death was reduced by 24% and 30%, respectively, in the cholestyramine group, that of all-cause mortality was reduced by only 7% (Table 3), reflecting an increase in deaths not caused by CHD. Table 5, patterned after a similar table reported in the World Health Organization Clofibrate Trial,[11] breaks down the all-cause mortality into major categories. None of the differences are statistically significant. More details are provided in Appendix B. The only noteworthy difference (P=.08) was 11 deaths from accidents and violence in the cholestyramine group, compared with four in the placebo group. Of these, five in the cholestyramine and two in the placebo group were homicides or suicides, and six in the cholestyramine and two in the placebo group were accidents, mainly automobile. Each of the other major categories, including malignant neoplasms, differed only by one or two cases.

The possibility that a CHD event

could have been the underlying cause of a violent or accidental death was examined. All of these deaths had been evaluated by the Cardiovascular Endpoints Committee without knowledge of treatment group, and none had met the study criteria of a CHD death. Furthermore, none had any clinical evidence suggestive of myocardial ischemia. Subsequent to the conclusion of the study, all of these deaths were carefully scrutinized for the possibility of a CHD event. Seven were due to homicide or suicide, and in none of these was there any reason to doubt the diagnosis. Autopsy information was available for seven of the eight accidental deaths; seven of these deaths were due to automobile or motorcycle accidents. None showed evidence of new coronary thrombosis or acute myocardial infarction. Half had high blood alcohol levels. In four, this information and the circumstances of death made it virtually certain that CHD was not an underlying cause of death. In the other four, although the circumstances of death did not completely rule it out, a CHD episode was regarded as highly unlikely.

### Possible Confounders

The results described previously show that the cholestyramine-treated group had a reduced rate of CHD. If during the course of the LRC-CPPT there were changes in CHD risk factors other than total cholesterol or LDL-C levels that were not the same in the two groups, this could pose an alternative explanation of the observed treatment benefit. Table 6 gives the pre-entry, first-year, and seventh-year mean values for selected variables that include the major known risk factors for CHD. For all of these major risk factors, the change from baseline was similar in the two groups, and, thus, they do not explain the treatment benefit. In addition, very similar percentages of participants in both groups (eg, placebo, 37%, v cholestyramine, 38%, at year 7) reported taking at least one aspirin in the previous week. Slightly more placebo- than cholestyramine-treated participants reported the use of β-blockers at the end of the trial.

### Side Effects and Toxicity

Many possible side effects to treatment were monitored throughout the

Table 5.—Deaths in the Lipid Research Clinics Coronary Primary Prevention Trial

| Cause of Death | Placebo | Cholestyramine Resin |
|---|---|---|
| Coronary heart disease (CHD) | 44 | 32 |
| Other vascular | 3 | 5 |
| Malignant neoplasm | 15 | 16 |
| Other medical causes | 5 | 4 |
| Accidents and violence | 4 | 11 |
| Total, all causes other than CHD | 27 | 36 |
| All causes other than CHD, other vascular, and accidents and violence | 20 | 20 |
| Total, all causes | 71 | 68 |

Table 8.—Selected Variables Before and During Treatment

| Variable | Placebo | | | Cholestyramine Resin | | |
|---|---|---|---|---|---|---|
| | Pre-entry | 1st Year | 7th Year | Pre-entry | 1st Year | 7th Year |
| Mean systolic blood pressure, mm Hg | 121 | 120 | 122 | 121 | 120 | 122 |
| Mean diastolic blood pressure, mm Hg | 80 | 79 | 78 | 80 | 78 | 78 |
| Mean Quetelet index, g/sq cm | 2.6 | 2.6 | 2.7 | 2.6 | 2.6 | 2.7 |
| Mean weight, kg | 81 | 81 | 83 | 80 | 80 | 82 |
| % current smokers | 37 | 35 | 26 | 38 | 36 | 27 |
| Mean cigarettes per day for current smokers | 25 | 24 | 25 | 26 | 25 | 26 |
| % regular exercisers | 30 | ...* | 27 | 31 | ...* | 28 |
| Median alcohol consumption, g/wk | 61 | 58 | 51 | 64 | 57 | 53 |

*No assessment of exercise was done in the first year.

trial. There were no noteworthy differences in non-GI side effects between the groups. Gastrointestinal side effects occurred frequently in the placebo- and cholestyramine-treated participants, especially the latter (Table 7). In the first year, 68% of the cholestyramine group experienced at least one GI side effect, compared with 43% of the placebo group. These diminished in frequency so that by the seventh year, approximately equal percentages of cholestyramine and placebo participants (29% v 26%) were so affected. Constipation and heartburn, especially, were more frequent in the cholestyramine group, which also reported more abdominal pain, belching or bloating, gas, and nausea. The side effects were usually not severe and could be dealt with by standard clinical means.

Little or no differences were seen between the two treatment groups for most of the clinical chemical tests monitored during the study (Appendix C). During the first year, serum alkaline phosphatase levels, iron binding capacity, SGOT levels, and the WBC count were higher in the cholestyramine group, while carotene and uric acid levels were lower (Table 8). These differences were generally less apparent by the seventh year; none was associated with clinically apparent disease.

The number of participants hospitalized for conditions other than CHD was monitored. The hospitalizations were classified, using the H-ICDA code, eighth revision,[19] according to the primary diagnosis on the hospital discharge form. In particular, hospitalizations for GI tract disease were monitored (Appendix D). Of the many categories, the only difference with nominal statistical significance, using a test of comparison of proportions, was the primary diagnosis of deviated nasal septum, with more (16 v 6) cases in the cholestyramine group. Similar monitoring of all noncardiac operations or procedures was conducted. The only significant difference was a greater number in the cholestyramine group (40 v 23) of operations or procedures involving the nervous system. This excess mainly reflected more operations or procedures in the cholestyramine group for spinal disease (23 v 10), especially lumbar (19 v 9), and for decompres-

sion of the carpal tunnel (7 v 1).

Diagnoses and procedures involving the gallbladder were scrutinized in view of the ability of certain lipid-lowering drugs to produce gallstones and gallbladder disease. A few more hospitalized participants in the cholestyramine group had, as their main diagnosis, gallstones (16 v 11) and more cholestyramine-treated participants had an operation involving the gallbladder (36 v 25), but the differences were not significant. Gallstones, not necessarily as the main diagnosis, were reported in the cholestyramine group slightly more frequently than in the placebo group (31 v 30), as were other gallbladder and biliary tract diseases (28 v 23). No death attributable to gallbladder disease was recorded.

Appendix E indicates that the numbers of incident and fatal cases of malignant neoplasms were similar in the two groups: 57 incident cases in the placebo group, of which 15 were fatal; and 57 incident cases in the cholestyramine group, of which 16 were fatal. The cholestyramine group had a few more malignant neoplasms in some categories (eg, buccal cavity and pharynx) and less in others (eg, respiratory system) than the placebo group, but the numbers were small. When the various categories of GI tract cancers (buccal cavity-pharynx, esophagus, stomach, colon, rectum, and pancreas) were considered together, there were 11 incident cases and one fatal case in the placebo group and 21 incident and eight fatal cases in the cholestyramine group. The total number of incident colon cancers was identical.

## COMMENT
### Previous Trials of Cholesterol Lowering

The LRC-CPPT demonstrated that treatment with cholestyramine resin reduced the incidence of CHD. This result is in agreement with those of previous clinical trials of cholesterol lowering, which have shown a general trend of efficacy for selected CHD end points. However, the earlier trials have not been regarded as conclusive because of such factors as inadequate sample size, absence of a double-blind, failure to achieve identical treatment groups, inadequate cholesterol lowering, or questionable statis-

| Table 7.—Percent of Participants Reporting Moderate or Severe Side Effects | | | | | | |
|---|---|---|---|---|---|---|
| | Placebo | | | Cholestyramine Resin | | |
| Side Effect | Pre-entry | 1st Year | 7th Year | Pre-entry | 1st Year | 7th Year |
| Abdominal pain | 5 | 11 | 7 | 5 | 15 | 7 |
| Belching or bloating | 10 | 18 | 6 | 10 | 27 | 9 |
| Constipation | 3 | 10 | 4 | 4 | 39 | 8 |
| Diarrhea | 8 | 11 | 8 | 5 | 10 | 4 |
| Gas | 22 | 26 | 12 | 22 | 32 | 12 |
| Heartburn | 10 | 10 | 7 | 10 | 27 | 12 |
| Nausea | 4 | 8 | 4 | 3 | 16 | 3 |
| Vomiting | 2 | 5 | 3 | 2 | 8 | 2 |
| At least 1 gastrointestinal side effect | 34 | 43 | 28 | 34 | 68 | 29 |

| Table 8.—Mean Laboratory Values Influenced by Cholestyramine Resin | | | | | | |
|---|---|---|---|---|---|---|
| | Placebo | | | Cholestyramine Resin | | |
| Laboratory Value | Pre-entry | 1st Year | 7th Year | Pre-entry | 1st Year | 7th Year |
| Alkaline phosphatase, IU/L of serum | 71 | 70 | 71 | 71 | 82 | 74 |
| Carotene, µg/dL of serum | 150 | 146 | 149 | 149 | 111 | 132 |
| Iron-binding capacity, µg/dL of serum | 355 | 355 | 324 | 357 | 371 | 334 |
| SGOT, units/L of serum | 30 | 31 | 35 | 30 | 34 | 38 |
| Uric acid, mg/dL of serum | 6.3 | 6.1 | 6.3 | 6.2 | 5.8 | 6.1 |
| WBC count, per cu mm | 6,205 | 6,178 | 6,043 | 6,327 | 6,443 | 6,299 |

tical procedures.[20,21]

Several major primary prevention trials of diet have reported encouraging, although not always significant, reductions in CHD incidence. They include the New York Anti-Coronary Club Study,[22] the Los Angeles Veterans Administration Study,[23] and the Finnish Mental Hospital Study.[24] The interpretation of the results of these studies, as well as secondary prevention studies using diet, is clouded by the ascertainment bias that may result from a nonblinded design. Because of this and other shortcomings, these trials have also been regarded as inconclusive.[21] Primary prevention of CHD by diet has been evaluated during concurrent reduction of other CHD risk factors. A 47% lower CHD incidence was observed in the hypercholesterolemic participants in the Oslo Study who were treated with a cholesterol-lowering diet and counseled to reduce their cigarette smoking.[25] The investigators attributed most of the lower CHD incidence to the cholesterol reduction. The Multiple Risk Factor Intervention Trial (MRFIT) achieved too small an overall difference (2%) between the cholesterol levels of its two treatment groups to assess the effect of cholesterol lowering.[26]

One major primary prevention trial of a lipid-lowering drug has been reported: the WHO Clofibrate Study obtained a 9% fall in serum cholesterol levels and a significant 20% reduction in the overall incidence of major ischemic heart disease events, similar in magnitude to the LRC-CPPT findings.[11] However, unlike the LRC-CPPT, this decline was confined to nonfatal myocardial infarction, whereas the incidence of fatal heart attack was similar in both treatment and control groups. Of concern in this study was the increased incidence in all-cause mortality in the clofibrate group, which became more significant during a four-year posttrial follow-up.[18,27]

The Coronary Drug Project (CDP) was a major secondary prevention trial of several lipid-lowering drugs. Three of its groups (high-dose estrogen, low-dose estrogen, and d-thyroxine) had to be discontinued prematurely because of evidence of toxicity.[28-30] The nicotinic acid group, in which a 9.9% fall in cholesterol levels occurred, showed a 27% lower incidence of nonfatal myocardial infarction but little difference in fatal CHD.[31] The clofibrate group, in which

a 6.5% reduction in cholesterol levels occurred, had a 9% lower incidence of fatal and nonfatal CHD, but statistical significance was not attained.[31] Two trials of clofibrate, the Newcastle Study[32] and the Scottish Society of Physicians Study,[33] had previously reported a suggestion of benefit, especially in subjects with pre-existing angina, but the post hoc use of subgroups and discordance in placebo group events has led to questioning of the conclusions from these two studies.[34]

The results of these various studies of lipid-lowering drugs for the prevention of CHD indicate that even though some evidence of reduction of CHD has attended their use, noteworthy and sometimes serious toxicity has occurred for each drug.

### Side Effects and Clinical Chemistry Analyses

The use of cholestyramine resin resulted in several GI side effects, although these were also common in the placebo group. They were most evident in the initial stages of the study and could usually be handled by symptom-specific treatment, but sometimes they were the basis for cessation of, or reduction in, the drug dose. These side effects, which have been previously noted for cholestyramine resin, reflect the properties of a drug that is not metabolized in, or absorbed from, the GI tract. The monitoring of hospitalizations showed that the two treatment groups were similar for almost all of the large number of primary diagnoses and procedures. Of special interest is the absence of a significant increase in gallstones or cholecystectomy. This contrasts with clofibrate, which, unlike cholestyramine resin, is known to alter the lithogenicity of bile and has been associated in the WHO and CDP trials with an increased incidence of gallbladder disease.[18,31] The results of a systematic radiological study for gallstones in participants at two LRCs before and after the LRC-CPPT will be published.

A greater incidence of respiratory system hospitalizations and operations and procedures on the nervous system was observed in the cholestyramine group. However, examination of the individual diagnoses or procedures within these categories failed to reveal any disorder for which there was a plausible explanation of an effect that could be attributed to cholestyramine resin. In view of the more than 60 diagnoses and procedures assessed, the two categories in which significant differences were found may represent chance occurrences.

Cholestyramine treatment altered results of several clinical chemistry studies, especially alkaline phosphatase, SGOT, and carotene. Such changes have been previously reported for cholestyramine use and, as in the present study, have not been associated with clinical disease.[5]

### Malignant Neoplasms

The total incidence of fatal and nonfatal malignant neoplasms was similar in both treatment groups. When the many different categories are examined, various GI tract cancers were somewhat more prevalent in the cholestyramine group. Other cancers (eg, lung and prostate) were more frequent in the placebo group. The small numbers and the multiple categories prevent conclusions being drawn. However, in view of the fact that cholestyramine resin is confined to the GI tract and not absorbed and of animal experiments in which cholestyramine resin has been found to be a promoter of colon cancer when a cancer-inducing agent was also fed orally,[35] further follow-up of the LRC-CPPT participants is planned for cause-specific mortality and cancer morbidity.

### CHD End Points

The LRC-CPPT shows that treatment with cholestyramine resin results in a significantly lower incidence of CHD as measured by the primary end point of the study. The benefit of treatment was not concentrated in any one subgroup or in a few clinics but was widespread. Inspection of the life-table curves shows that benefit became apparent two years after initial treatment. This benefit was reflected in both categories of primary end points. The findings were not essentially altered when the men classified as having a "suspect" primary event were added to the definite CHD category, nor were they altered by the inclusion of

the small number of intraoperative events in the primary end-point category. The possibility was considered that some deaths attributed to violence or accidents were precipitated by a CHD event, especially since more of them occurred in the cholestyramine group. As described, an extensive review of autopsy and clinical evidence was convincing that it was extremely unlikely that an underlying CHD event had occurred in any of the accidental or violent deaths.

The evidence of reduction of CHD incidence is further strongly supported by the analysis of other CHD end points for which a sufficient number occurred. Other studies have reported that angina and a positive exercise test result identify subjects at increased risk for CHD. In the LRC-CPPT, angina at entry was an exclusion. A positive exercise test result at entry, in the absence of chest pain, was a significant independent predictor of a subsequent primary end point, using proportional hazards analysis (to be published). Thus, the development of angina or new positive exercise test results, although not primary study end points, seem to be valid indicators of CHD risk status. Incident cases of the development of angina or of a new positive exercise test result were substantially lower by 20% and 25%, respectively, in the cholestyramine group. A corresponding 21% reduction was observed in the number of participants progressing to coronary bypass surgery. Also of interest is the 15% reduction in intermittent claudication.

### All-Cause Mortality

There was only a 7% reduction of all-cause mortality in the cholestyramine group, reflecting a larger number of violent and accidental deaths. Several other primary prevention trials have reported higher noncardiovascular mortality in their active treatment groups, resulting from a variety of medical causes.[36] Excess mortality in the LRC-CPPT cholestyramine group was confined to violent and accidental deaths. Since no plausible connection could be established between cholestyramine treatment and violent or accidental death, it is difficult to conclude that this could be anything but a chance occurrence.

### Confounding

The lower incidence in CHD events seen in the cholestyramine group does not seem to be attributable to changes in CHD risk factors other than cholesterol. The use of randomization and stratification procedures produced two treatment groups that, at entry, were similar with respect to all the major CHD risk factors, other minor or possible risk factors, and a variety of other measurements. The levels of CHD risk factors such as cigarette smoking, systolic and diastolic blood pressure, body weight, and reported levels of physical activity continued to be similar throughout the study. Both groups reported similar nutrient intakes and alcohol consumption.

### Maintenance of Double-Blind

Many steps were taken to ensure that neither participants nor clinic staff knew to which treatment group participants had been assigned.[1] No need arose during the study to identify a participant's treatment group to him or to clinical staff. The higher incidence of GI effects in the cholestyramine group, mainly in the first year, made it possible that some loss of the double-blind might have occurred, although the high prevalence of such side effects in the placebo group makes this less likely. A survey at the end of the study showed that approximately equal numbers of participants (cholestyramine group, 56.0% v placebo group, 54.6%) or clinic staff (cholestyramine group, 55.2% v placebo group, 52.9%) could correctly identify treatment assignments.

### Implementation of Study Design

The extent to which the LRC-CPPT was able to implement its original design objectives[1] is noteworthy (Table 9). The study exceeded its original sample size goal of 3,550 and successfully randomized 3,806 participants into two similar treatment groups. Participants were followed up for an average of 7.4 years. Consistent with the initial study parameters, a 4.8% reduction in plasma total cholesterol levels attributed to diet was obtained in the placebo group. In the seventh year, men taking cholestyramine resin maintained a mean plasma total cholesterol level reduction of 13.9%, attributable to the combination of drug and diet. Thus, the additional reduction in cholesterol levels attributable to cholestyramine resin was only 9.1%, well below the desired 24%. Although the 27% of participants who were taking no drug by seven years was lower than the predicted 35%, a number of participants were not taking the full dose of six packets. Difficulties in adherence related to the bulk, texture, and side effects of the drug seem to explain much of the shortfall in cholesterol lowering. It can be effectively argued that additional deterrents to taking the drug were the participants' lack of knowledge, for seven to ten years, as to which treatment group they were in as well as of their cholesterol levels during treatment. Better cholesterol lowering with cholestyramine resin could be expected when it is used in a routine clinical context. In addition, knowledge that treatment with cholestyramine resin prevents CHD can be expected to motivate adherence.

The seven-year incidence of the combined primary end points in the LRC-CPPT placebo group, 8.6%, was almost identical to the 8.7% predicted in the original study design based on data derived from the Framingham Study.[17] However, the actual incidence of definite CHD death was well below the predicted rate, whereas the rate of definite nonfatal myocardial infarction was increased above the predicted rate. A lower-than-predicted CHD death rate has been a feature of several clinical trials, including the recent MRFIT study.[36] Possible explanations include the stringent selection processes employed, resulting in an atypically healthier study population, better health monitoring and management during the course of the study, and the concurrent national decline in CHD mortality.

### Implications of the LRC-CPPT

Caution should be exercised before extrapolating the CPPT findings to cholesterol-lowering drugs other than bile acid sequestrants. It has been shown that bile acid sequestration leads to a substantial reduction in plasma total and LDL-C levels by increasing the removal of LDL from the blood through increased activity

of specific cell-surface LDL receptors.[14] This mode of action is conceptually attractive inasmuch as it represents the enhancement of a physiological mechanism for the control of LDL levels. The mode of action, cholesterol-lowering potency, and possible toxicity of other cholesterol-lowering drugs must be taken into account before their use is advocated for the prevention of CHD.

The LRC-CPPT was not designed to assess directly whether cholesterol lowering by diet prevents CHD. Nevertheless, its findings, taken in conjunction with the large volume of evidence relating diet, plasma cholesterol levels, and CHD, support the view that cholesterol lowering by diet also would be beneficial. The findings of the LRC-CPPT take on additional significance if it is acknowledged that it is unlikely that a conclusive study of dietary-induced cholesterol lowering for the prevention of CHD can be designed or implemented.

The consistency of the reductions in CHD manifestations observed with cholestyramine resin in this controlled trial, which extend from the softer end points of angina, a positive exercise test result, and coronary bypass surgery to the hard end points of nonfatal myocardial infarction and CHD death, leaves little doubt of the benefit of cholestyramine therapy. These results could be narrowly interpreted to apply only to the use of bile acid sequestrants in middle-aged men with cholesterol levels above 265 mg/dL (perhaps 1 to 2 million Americans). The trial's implications, however, could and should be extended to other age groups and women and, since cholesterol levels and CHD risk are continuous variables, to others

with more modest elevations of cholesterol levels. The benefits that could be expected from cholestyramine treatment are considerable. In the LRC-CPPT, treatment was associated with an average cholesterol fall of 8.5% beyond diet, and an average 19% reduction in CHD risk. Moreover, a companion article[17] that looks at cholesterol reduction and CHD more closely indicates that a 49% reduction in CHD incidence would be predicted for subjects who obtained a 25% fall in plasma cholesterol levels or a 35% fall in LDL-C levels, which are typical responses to 24 g of cholestyramine resin daily.

Funding for the study came from the following National Heart, Lung, and Blood Institute contracts and interagency agreements: N01-HV1-2156-L, N01-HV1-2160-L, N01-HV2-2914-L, N01-HV3-2931-L, Y01-HV3-0010-L, N01-HV2-2913-L, N01-HV1-2158-L, N01-HV1-2161-L, N01-HV2-2915-L, N01-HV2-2932-L, N01-HV2-2917-L, N01-HV2-2916-L, N01-HV1-2157-L, N01-HV1-2243-L, N01-HV1-2159-L, N01-HV3-2961-L, and N01-HV6-2941-L.

The Lipid Research Clinics Program acknowledges the long-term commitment of the volunteer participants in this clinical trial.

Lipid Research Clinics Coronary Primary Prevention Trial sites and key personnel are listed as follows.

**Lipid Research Clinics**

Baylor College of Medicine, Houston
Principal investigator: William Insull, MD; associate director (former principal investigator): Antonio M. Gotto, MD, PhD; CPPT director: Jeffrey Probstfield, MD; former CPPT directors: O. David Taunton, MD, Ellison Wittels, MD; key personnel: Susan Andrews, MA, Mohammed Attar, MD, Katherine Canizares, Janice Henske, MPH, RD, Tsai-Lien Lin, MS, Wolfgang Patsch, MD, Georgia White, RN.
University of Cincinnati Medical Center
Principal investigator: Charles J. Glueck, MD; CPPT director: Jane Third, MD; former CPPT directors: Ronald Fallat, MD, Moti Kashyap, MD, Evan Stein, MD; key personnel: Robert Adolph, MD, W. Fraser Bremner, MD, Jack Friedel, PhD, Rhea Larsen, RD, Susan McNeeley, MS, Paula Steiner, MS.

Table 9.—Comparison of LRC-CPPT* Design Goals and Actual Experience

| Design Feature | Goal | Experience |
| --- | --- | --- |
| Sample size | 3,550 | 3,806† |
| Duration of follow-up, yr | 7 | 7-10 |
| Lost to follow-up | 0 | 0 |
| Reduction of plasma total cholesterol levels in placebo group | 4% | 4.8% |
| Nonadherers‡ at yr 7 | 35% | 27% |
| Reduction of plasma total cholesterol levels in men adhering‡ to cholestyramine resin treatment | 28% | 13.9%§ |
| 7-yr incidence of primary end point in placebo group | 8.7% | 8.8% |
| Reduction in primary end point | 38% | 19% |

*LRC-CPPT indicates Lipid Research Clinics Coronary Primary Prevention Trial.
†After removal of four type III participants.
‡A nonadherer is someone averaging less than half a packet of cholestyramine resin per day.
§Computed for seventh year.

### References

1. Levy RI: Review: Declining mortality in coronary heart disease. Arteriosclerosis 1981; 1:312-325.
2. Gordon T, Castelli WP, Hjortland MC, et al: The prediction of coronary heart disease by high-density and other lipoproteins: An historical perspective, in Rifkind B, Levy R (eds): Hyperlipidemia—Diagnosis and Therapy. New York, Grune & Stratton Inc, 1977, pp 71-78.
3. Stamler J: Population studies, in Levy RI, Rifkind RM, Dennis BH, et al (eds): Nutrition, Lipids, and Coronary Heart Disease. New York, Raven Press, 1979, pp 25-88.
4. Arteriosclerosis: A Report by the National Heart and Lung Institute Task Force on Arteriosclerosis. Dept of Health, Education, and Welfare publication (NIH) 72-137. Washington, DC, National Institutes of Health, 1971, vol 1.
5. Levy RI, Fredrickson DS, Stone NJ, et al: Cholestyramine in type II hyperlipoproteinemia: A double-blind trial. Ann Intern Med 1973; 79:51-58.

6. The Lipid Research Clinics Program: The Coronary Primary Prevention Trial: Design and implementation. J Chronic Dis 1979;32:609-631.
7. Protocol for the Lipid Research Clinics Type II Coronary Primary Prevention Trial. Chapel Hill, NC, University of North Carolina Department of Biostatistics, 1980.
8. The Lipid Research Clinics Program: Participant recruitment to the Coronary Primary Prevention Trial. J Chronic Dis 1983;36:451-465.
9. The Lipid Research Clinics Program: Recruitment for clinical trials: The Lipid Research Clinics Coronary Primary Prevention Trial experience. Circulation 1982;66(suppl 4):1-78.
10. The Lipid Research Clinics Program: Pre-entry characteristics of participants in the Lipid Research Clinics Coronary Primary Prevention Trial. J Chronic Dis 1983;36:467-479.
11. Dennis B, Ernst N, Hjortland M, et al: The NHLBI nutrition data system. J Am Diet Assoc 1980;77:641-647.
12. Kalbfleisch JD, Prentice RL: The Statisti-

cal Analysis of Failure Time Data. New York, John Wiley & Sons, 1980.
13. O'Brien PC, Fleming TR: A multiple testing procedure for clinical trials. Biometrics 1979;35:549-556.
14. Majundar H, Sen PK: Nonparametric testing for simple linear regression under progressive censoring with staggering entry and random withdrawal. Communication in Statistics—Theory and Methods 1978;A7:349-371.
15. Breslow N, Haug C: Sequential comparison of exponential survival curves. J Am Stat Assoc 1972;67:691-697.
16. Tsiatis AA: The asymptomatic joint distributions of efficient scores test for the proportional hazards model over time. Biometrika 1981;68:311-315.
17. Lipid Research Clinics Program: The Lipid Research Clinics Coronary Primary Prevention Trial Results: II. The relationship of reduction in incidence of coronary heart disease to cholesterol lowering. JAMA 1984;251:365-374.

18. Committee of Principal Investigators, W.H.O. Clofibrate Trial: A cooperative trial in the primary prevention of ischaemic heart disease using clofibrate, report. *Br Heart J* 1978; 40:1069-1118.

19. *H-ICDA: Hospital Adaptation of ICDA*, ed 2, eighth revision. Ann Arbor, Mich, Commission on Professional and Hospital Activities, 1973, vol 1.

20. Cornfield J, Mitchell S: Selected risk factors in coronary disease: Possible intervention effects. *Arch Environ Health* 1969;19:382-391.

21. Davis CE, Havlik R: Clinical trials of lipid lowering and coronary artery disease prevention, in Rifkind BM, Levy RI (eds): *Hyperlipidemia—Diagnosis and Therapy*. New York, Grune & Stratton Inc, 1977, pp 79-92.

22. Rinzler SH: Primary prevention of coronary heart disease by diet. *Bull NY Acad Med* 1968;44:936-949.

23. Dayton S, Pearce ML, Hashimoto S, et al: A controlled clinical trial of a diet high in unsaturated fat in preventing complications of atherosclerosis. *Circulation* 1969;39-40(suppl 2):1-63.

24. Turpeinen O, Karvonen MJ, Pekkarinen M, et al: Dietary prevention of coronary heart disease: The Finnish Mental Hospital Study. *Int J Epidemiol* 1979;8:99-118.

25. Hjermann I, Velve Byre K, Holme I, et al: Effect of diet and smoking intervention on the incidence of coronary heart disease: Report from the Oslo Study Group of a randomized trial in healthy men. *Lancet* 1981;2:1303-1310.

26. Multiple Risk Factor Intervention Trial Research Group: Multiple Risk Factor Intervention Trial: Risk factor changes and mortality results. *JAMA* 1982;248:1465-1477.

27. Committee of Principal Investigators, W.H.O. Clofibrate Trial: W.H.O. Cooperative Trial on primary prevention of ischaemic heart disease using clofibrate to lower serum cholesterol: Mortality follow-up report. *Lancet* 1980; 2:379-385.

28. Coronary Drug Project Research Group: The Coronary Drug Project: Initial findings leading to modification of its research protocol. *JAMA* 1970;214:1303-1313.

29. Coronary Drug Project Research Group: The Coronary Drug Project: Findings leading to discontinuation of the 2.5 mg/day estrogen group. *JAMA* 1973;226:652-657.

30. Coronary Drug Project Research Group: The Coronary Drug Project: Findings leading to further modifications of its protocol with respect to dextrothyroxine. *JAMA* 1972;220:996-1008.

31. Coronary Drug Project Research Group: The Coronary Drug Project: Clofibrate and niacin in coronary heart disease. *JAMA* 1975; 231:360-381.

32. Group of Physicians of the Newcastle Upon Tyne Region: Trial of clofibrate in the treatment of ischaemic heart disease: Five-year study. *Br Med J* 1971;4:767-775

33. Research Committee of the Scottish Society of Physicians: Ischaemic heart disease: A secondary prevention trial using clofibrate. *Br Med J* 1971;4:775-784.

34. Friedewald WT, Halperin M: Clofibrate in ischemic heart disease. *Ann Intern Med* 1972; 76:821-823.

35. Asano T, Pollard M, Madsen DC: Effects of cholestyramine on 1,2-dimethylhydrazine-induced enteric carcinoma in germfree rats. *Proc Soc Exp Biol Med* 1975;150:780-785.

36. Oliver MF: Serum cholesterol: The knave of hearts and the joker. *Lancet* 1981;2:1090-1095.

37. Kannel WB, Castelli WP, Gordon T, et al: Serum cholesterol, lipoproteins and the risk of coronary heart disease: The Framingham Study. *Ann Intern Med* 1971;74:1-12.

38. Goldstein JL, Kita T, Brown MS: Defective lipoprotein receptors and atherosclerosis: Lessons from an animal counterpart of familial hypercholesterolemia. *N Engl J Med* 1983; 309:288-296.

39. Blackburn H, Keys A, Simonson E, et al: The electrocardiogram in population study. *Circulation* 1960;21:1160-1175.

---

**Appendix A.—Definition of Primary End Points**

**Primary End Points**

I. Definite atherosclerotic coronary heart disease death—either or both of the following categories:

  A. Death certificate with consistent underlying or immediate cause plus either of the following:

    1. Preterminal hospitalization with definite or suspect myocardial infarction (see below).

    2. Previous definite angina or suspect or definite myocardial infarction when no cause other than atherosclerotic coronary heart disease could be ascribed as the cause of death.

  B. Sudden and unexpected death (requires all three characteristics):

    1. Deaths occurring within one hour after the onset of severe symptoms or having last been seen without them.

    2. No known nonatherosclerotic acute or chronic process or event that could have been potentially lethal.

    3. An "unexpected" death occurs only in a person who is not confined to his home, hospital, or other institution because of illness within 24 hours before death.

II. Criteria for definite nonfatal myocardial infarction—any one or more of the following categories using the stated definitions:

  A. Diagnostic ECG at the time of the event.

  B. Ischemic cardiac pain and diagnostic enzymes.

  C. Ischemic cardiac pain and equivocal enzymes and equivocal ECG.

  D. A routine Lipid Research Clinics ECG is diagnostic for myocardial infarction while the previous one was not.

III. Suspect atherosclerotic coronary heart disease death—one or both of the following categories:

  A. Death certificate with consistent underlying or immediate cause but neither adequate preterminal documentation of the event nor previous atherosclerotic coronary heart disease diagnosis.

  B. Rapid and unexpected death (requires all three characteristics):

    1. Death occurring between one and 24 hours after the onset of severe symptoms or having last been seen without them.

    2. No known nonatherosclerotic acute or chronic process or event that could have been potentially lethal.

    3. An "unexpected death" occurs only in a person who is not confined to his home, hospital, or other institution because of illness within 24 hours before death.

IV. Suspect myocardial infarction—any one or more of the following categories using the stated definitions:

  A. Ischemic cardiac pain.

  B. Diagnostic enzymes.

  C. Equivocal ECG and equivocal enzymes.

  D. Equivocal ECG alone, provided that it is not based on ST or T-wave changes only.

*(Continued on page 363.)*

Appendix A.—Definition of Primary End Points (cont)

**Glossary**

I. Ischemic cardiac pain—severe substernal pain having a deep or visceral quality and lasting for half an hour or more.

II. ECG (classified by Minnesota Code)[38]

  A. Diagnostic—either of the following must be present:

    1. Unequivocal Q or QS pattern (code 1-1).

    2. Q or QS pattern (codes 1-2-1 to 1-2-7), plus any T-wave item (codes 5-1 to 5-3).

    Only the first criterion applies in the presence of ventricular conduction defects.

  B. Equivocal—any of the following must be present:

    1. Q or QS pattern (codes 1-2-1 to 1-2-7).

    2. ST junction and segment depression (codes 4-1 to 4-3).

    3. T-wave item (codes 5-1 to 5-2).

    4. Left bundle-branch block (code 7-1).

III. Enzymes

  A. Diagnostic enzymes—all of the following conditions:

    1. Creatine kinase, SGOT, or lactic dehydrogenase values determined coexistent with the event.

    2. The upper limit of normal for the local laboratory is recorded.

    3. The determined value for one or more enzymes is at least twice the upper limit of the local laboratory but does not exceed 15 times that value.

  B. Equivocal enzymes—all of the following conditions:

    1. Creatine kinase, SGOT, or lactic dehydrogenase values determined coexistent with the event.

    2. The upper limit of normal for the local laboratory is recorded.

    3. The determined value for one or more enzymes is elevated but does not fulfill criteria for diagnostic enzymes.

Appendix B.—Deaths Not Attributed to Coronary Heart Disease

| Cause of Death | Placebo | Cholestyramine Resin |
|---|---|---|
| Cardiovascular (non-coronary heart disease) | 3 | 5 |
| Cerebrovascular | 2 | 2 |
| Peripheral vascular with gangrene | 0 | 1 |
| Surgical complications* | 1 | 2 |
| Malignant neoplasm† | 15 | 16 |
| Other illnesses | 5 | 4 |
| Infectious diseases‡ | 3 | 2 |
| Chronic obstructive pulmonary disease | 1 | 1 |
| Alcoholism | 1 | 1 |
| Trauma | 4 | 11 |
| Accidents | 2 | 6 |
| Homicide | 0 | 1 |
| Suicide | 2 | 4 |
| Total | 27 | 36 |

*One placebo participant died while undergoing cardiac catheterization. Two cholestyramine resin participants died of complications ensuing from mitral valve replacement and from carotid endarterectomy.

†Listed by site in Appendix E.

‡Three deaths (two in the placebo group) caused by pneumonia, one placebo death caused by staphylococcal septicemia, and one cholestyramine resin death resulting from an undetermined infectious cause.

### Appendix C.—Mean Laboratory Values Not Influenced by Cholestyramine Resin

| Laboratory Value | Placebo | | | Cholestyramine Resin | | |
|---|---|---|---|---|---|---|
| | Pre-entry | 1st Year | 7th Year | Pre-entry | 1st Year | 7th Year |
| Albumin, g/dL of serum | 4.3 | 4.2 | 4.2 | 4.3 | 4.2 | 4.2 |
| Bilirubin, direct, mg/dL of serum | 0.04 | 0.04 | 0.04 | 0.04 | 0.05 | 0.04 |
| Bilirubin, total, mg/dL of serum | 0.52 | 0.52 | 0.61 | 0.52 | 0.54 | 0.62 |
| Calcium, mEq/L of serum | 4.8 | 4.8 | 4.7 | 4.9 | 4.8 | 4.8 |
| Chloride, mEq/L of serum | 103 | 104 | 103 | 103 | 105 | 103 |
| Creatinine, mg/dL of serum | 1.03 | 1.02 | 0.98 | 1.03 | 1.01 | 0.98 |
| Globulin, g/dL of serum | 2.9 | 3.0 | 3.0 | 2.9 | 3.0 | 3.0 |
| Glucose, mg/dL of serum | 98 | 96 | 101 | 98 | 94 | 100 |
| Hematocrit, % | 46 | 45 | 45 | 46 | 45 | 45 |
| Iron, μg/dL of serum | 114 | 113 | 103 | 113 | 114 | 103 |
| Phosphorus, mg/dL of serum | 3.1 | 3.0 | 3.0 | 3.1 | 3.0 | 3.0 |
| Potassium, mEq/L of serum | 4.5 | 4.5 | 4.4 | 4.5 | 4.5 | 4.4 |
| Sodium, mEq/L of serum | 140 | 141 | 141 | 140 | 140 | 141 |
| Thyroxine, μg of $T_4$-I/dL of serum | 4.1 | 4.0 | 4.3 | 4.1 | 4.1 | 4.3 |
| Total protein, g/dL of serum | 7.2 | 7.2 | 7.3 | 7.2 | 7.2 | 7.3 |
| Vitamin A, IU/dL of serum | 228 | 234 | 267 | 229 | 236 | 270 |

### Appendix D.—Hospitalizations With a Primary Diagnosis[*] of Gastrointestinal Tract Disease

| Primary Diagnosis[†] | Placebo | Cholestyramine Resin |
|---|---|---|
| Intestinal infectious diseases | 13 | 9 |
| Neoplasm | | |
| Benign | 11 | 12 |
| Malignant | 11 | 15 |
| Unspecified | 0 | 1 |
| Diseases of esophagus | 5 | 6 |
| Ulcer | 20 | 30 |
| Gastritis | 5 | 12 |
| Functional and other disorders of stomach | 3 | 0 |
| Appendicitis | 4 | 11 |
| Hernia | 100 | 97 |
| Intestinal obstruction | 5 | 4 |
| Enteritis and colitis | 2 | 1 |
| Diverticular disease of intestine | 9 | 10 |
| Anal fissure and fistula | 9 | 5 |
| Abscess of anal and rectal region | 5 | 5 |
| Peritonitis | 0 | 1 |
| Functional and other diseases of intestine | 3 | 6 |
| Liver disease | 2 | 3 |
| Gallstones | 11 | 16 |
| Other gallbladder and biliary tract disease | 19 | 22 |
| Pancreas | 0 | 3 |
| Hemorrhoids | 27 | 29 |
| Signs, symptoms, and ill-defined conditions | 23 | 16 |

[*]Participants are counted only once within each category.
[†]By H-ICDA code, eighth revision, 1973.

### Appendix E.—Incident Malignant Neoplasms

| Primary Site | Placebo (N=1,900) | | Cholestyramine Resin (N=1,906) | |
|---|---|---|---|---|
| | All Cases | Deaths[*] | All Cases | Deaths[*] |
| Buccal cavity-pharynx | 0 | 0 | 6 | 0 |
| Esophagus | 1 | 0 | 2 | 2 |
| Stomach | 2 | 1 | 0 | 0 |
| Colon | 6 | 0 | 8 | 2 |
| Rectum | 2 | 0 | 4 | 1 |
| Pancreas | 0 | 0 | 3 | 3 |
| Larynx | 3 | 0 | 1 | 0 |
| Lung | 10 | 8 | 8 | 3 |
| Leiomyosarcoma | 1 | 1 | 0 | 0 |
| Melanoma | 5 | 1 | 0 | 0 |
| Other skin | 5 | 0 | 3 | 0 |
| Prostate | 11 | 1 | 7 | 1 |
| Urinary bladder | 3 | 0 | 7 | 0 |
| Kidney | 1 | 0 | 2 | 0 |
| Brain | 1 | 1 | 3 | 3 |
| Thyroid | 1 | 1 | 0 | 0 |
| Thymus | 0 | 0 | 1 | 0 |
| Lymphatic tissue | 1 | 0 | 4 | 1 |
| Hematopoietic tissue | 3 | 1 | 2 | 0 |
| Unknown | 1 | 0 | 1 | 0 |
| Total | 57 | 15 | 57[†] | 16 |

[*]Four men with malignant neoplasms (two in each treatment group) died of nonneoplastic causes. They are counted among the incident cases but not among the deaths in this Table.
[†]One cholestyramine group participant, who survived to the end of the study, had both a prostate carcinoma and a lymphoma; he is counted only once in the total.

How to Read and Interpret the LRC-CPPT Report

The abstract is given in bold type above the start of the narrative on the first page. The first few sentences describe the bare bones of the study. The middle part gives a brief summary of the results. Note here that other than the one sentence stating that the cumulative incidence for the primary end points were 8.6% and 7.0%, all results are given in terms of relative risk reduction rather than absolute risk reduction. For example, the reduction in coronary heart disease (CHD) deaths and nonfatal myocardial infarctions (NFMIs) are said to be 24% and 19%, respectively. The absolute risk reductions for these two outcomes were 0.4% and 1.5%. Using the relative risk figures is a common tactic employed to make insignificant differences appear much larger than they really are. But if the authors had used the latter figures, no one would take seriously their concluding statement about this study providing *strong* evidence for a causal role for total cholesterol and LDL cholesterol in CHD. In fact, this is not even strong evidence for an *association* between cholesterol and CHD, much less a causation.

The introductory section sets out first to place the study in context by describing the scope of the problem and the outcomes of prior investigations. The first paragraph gives the usual statements about CHD being the leading cause of death, greater than all forms of cancer, and so on. Because we know that the statistics are drawn from death certificates, which vastly inflates the incidence of heart disease, it is fair to say that these statements are overblown and self-serving. The truth is that we don't know the true incidence of death from CHD.

The second paragraph says that "The view that LDL-C is intimately involved in atherogenesis…is sustained" by many previous studies. This statement is simply false. There have been no studies that pass even minimal scientific muster that prove a causative role for LDL-C in atherosclerosis (AS).

The third paragraph concludes by stating that prior clinical trials of cholesterol lowering have been inconclusive. Of course, one could also say that inconclusive means the studies have shown no relationship between cholesterol lowering and CHD because there is none.

The fourth paragraph begins with a statement that can only be described as bizarre. The authors state, "the most appropriate clinical trial of the efficacy of cholesterol lowering would be a dietary study." They are so philosophically committed to the Diet-Heart Theory that they are unable to admit that a dietary study wasn't done because dietary change won't affect cholesterol levels very much, as demonstrated in many prior experiments. Thus, the paper's abstract and introduction contain many misleading and some outright false statements. They also summarize the data in a deceptive fashion. These findings should raise some suspicion about the scientific objectivity of the authors.

The next section of the paper is titled "Participants and Methods" and is the so-called nuts-and-bolts section. One of the reasons the selection process is important is that it defines the population to which the results may be applied. When the sample is drawn randomly from the general population, one may say that the results can be applied to the whole population, but when the sample is taken from a small slice of the population, one must be very cautious about extrapolating the results to the remainder of the population. The LRC study recruited healthy men between the ages of 35 and 59 with cholesterol levels greater than 265 mg/dl and no evidence of or prior history of heart disease. Because a cholesterol level above 265 mg/dl places the subjects above the 95th percentile of middle-aged men, this is a very narrow slice indeed. Because the theory is that high cholesterol equals high risk for CHD, it is understandable that the authors would want to test the efficacy of cholesterol lowering in the population at highest risk. If they wished to extrapolate the results to other segments of the population such as women or people with "normal" cholesterol levels, they should have included a few more experimental and control groups in the study. For example, it would have been easy to include a group with cholesterol levels in the lowest 10th or 20th percentiles. With all the clinics and experimental procedures already in place, the additional cost wouldn't have been excessive. It may be that the investigators were afraid of what this might reveal—that is, that those with low cholesterol levels might die and/or have heart attacks with about the same frequency as those with the highest cholesterol levels.

It is interesting that in spite of the claim that those with evidence of CHD were excluded, the study *included* men with positive exercise tests. Those subjects with symptoms of angina pectoris (chest pain) were excluded even though chest pain is somewhat subjective in its perception and evaluation. However, positive exercise tests in males have been shown to be about 80% reliable in identifying significant CHD in the absence of symptoms. Obviously, the investigators were aware of this, because they list "positive exercise test" along with angina pectoris among the "other cardiovascular endpoints" in the results section of the paper. As long as the subjects with the positive exercise tests were evenly distributed between the experimental and control groups, it would not affect the outcome of the study. However, it would be interesting to know how many of the cardiac deaths and heart attacks came from this group, as that would further narrow the applicability of the results. Unfortunately, we are given no data on either of these two questions.

Although patient selection is important, the real key in this section is how the data are collected and evaluated. Although they are not crucial to this study, the dietary data deserve some comment. The authors tell us that a 24-hour dietary recall was elicited from each subject semiannually. This means that twice a year, the subjects reported on the foods and the quantities eaten over the previous 24 hours. The investigators then estimated the caloric intake, percentage as fat, etc. Subjects' dietary intake *for the whole year* was then based on these two recalls. That is, their total calories, percent of calories as fat, ratio of saturated fat to unsaturated fat, cholesterol intake, and so on, were all assumed to be faithfully reflected in two 24-hour recalls. Even though it has been shown time and again that most people will "fudge" their responses to appear less self-indulgent or to more closely approximate the perceived desires of the investigator, these and other authors of dietary studies continue to rely on such imprecise methods. Of course, only our most highly educated scholars would accept this kind of data as accurate. The average person with common sense would be amazed to learn that this type of "data" is the basis for most dietary studies that are quoted in the press.

But because diet isn't really the focus of this clinical trial, let's zero in on the data that really matter. What are the end points, how are they defined, and, most important, how were they assigned to the individual cases? The primary end point chosen was the combination of death due to CHD and NFMIs. As mentioned previously, because of the inherent inaccuracies in assessing cause of death and the occurrence of myocardial infarction (MI), these are both relatively soft end points and combining those does nothing to "harden" them. The authors, however, have enough confidence in their definitions and procedures to label some as definite CHD death and definite NFMI as opposed to suspected CHD deaths or NFMIs. The criteria and definitions are given in their Appendix A.

The authors' definitions of primary end points tells us that definite CHD death may be diagnosed based on *either* a death certificate diagnosis with some minor corroborative evidence *or* a sudden and unexpected death. The latter is qualified by requiring three additional characteristics, but careful reading of the language shows that virtually *any* sudden death would qualify. The criteria for definite NFMI include "ischemic cardiac pain" (a very subjective sign or symptom) and "equivocal enzymes and equivocal ECG." This alone is enough to invalidate the data for NFMI. It seems to stretch the language beyond the limits of rationality to claim that equivocal diagnostic data can lead to a definite diagnostic classification. Because we know that the error rate for death certificates, cause of sudden death, and diagnosis of MI can be as high as 30%–50%, it is not reasonable to categorize these end points as hard. Perhaps the inaccuracies would cancel each other out if the different groups were large enough, but as we shall see when we get to the results, the numbers are so small that only a few misdiagnoses would be enough to invert the results.

The only hard end point in the study is total mortality (all causes), and it is relegated to the status of a secondary end point. Of course, including it as a primary end point would have rendered the entire study insignificant even by the rather lax criteria of significance adopted here.

The final part of the Methods section concerns statistical methods. If your eyes glaze over when reading the names of the esoteric statistical techniques employed, do not despair. This entire discussion can be ignored, for we will seek out the pertinent raw data, calculate simple percentages, and apply common sense to determine significance.

The Results section is where we will find these numbers. In this study, the pertinent data can be found in Table 3. Because the authors almost never mention the absolute risk reduction but instead always give the more impressive-sounding relative risk reduction, it is helpful to construct your own table with the relevant numbers. For this study, that table would look like this:

| | Placebo | | Cholestyramine | | Absolute RR |
|---|---|---|---|---|---|
| | No | % | No | % | |
| 1. Total Mortality | 71 | 3.7 | 68 | 3.6 | 0.1% |
| 2. CHD deaths | 38 | 2.0 | 30 | 1.6 | 0.4% |
| 3. NFMIs | 158 | 8.3 | 130 | 6.8 | 1.5% |
| 4. Combined CHD deaths & NFMIs* | 87 | 9.8 | 155 | 8.1 | 1.7% |

*Note that the sum of the numbers on lines two and three does not add up to the same number that is on line four. This is because several patients suffered a NFMI and later died from CHD.

When the figures are presented honestly like this, it is obvious that the differences are miniscule, which explains why the authors only present the results in terms of relative risk reduction. Take, for example, the category of "Definite CHD Deaths." As we have seen, this diagnosis is subject to considerable error, and here, a misdiagnosis of only four cases would erase the difference entirely.

Of course, the way the results are presented speaks volumes about the agenda of the authors. We have already seen that they never give the absolute risk reduction figures in either the narrative description or in the tables. They describe a reduction in total mortality (the only hard end point) as "only 7%" and never mention that the absolute risk reduction was 0.1% (one-tenth of one percent). They also fail to mention that the difference in total mortality between the treatment and control groups is statistically insignificant by any test. Common sense tells us that none of the differences seen in our table are of any practical significance no matter what statistical sleight of hand is applied to make them appear otherwise.

The authors also present the data on a graph labeled "Life Table Cumulative Incidence of Primary End Points." It is important to realize that this is simply a graphic representation over time of the same two relatively soft end points that comprise the primary end point. The authors claim that after the second year, there was a "steady divergence of the two sets of event rates"; the implication is that the two lines would continue to separate further over time. This visual impression is particularly enhanced by the wider gap seen on the right edge of the graph. However, notice the huge drop-off in the number of subjects in the eighth and especially ninth years of follow-up. This would suggest that the numbers of events were so small as to render the differences insignificant. A second visual trick involves shortening the *y* axis. Note that the vertical *y* axis gives the cumulative percentage incidence ranging from 0% to 12%. If the same lines were plotted on a graph where the *y* axis was 0% to 100%, the two lines would appear to be almost superimposed on one another. This truncation of the *y* axis is a clever technique described by Darrell Huff in his classic work *How to Lie with Statistics*.

The other tables mostly give ancillary data and are not all that important to the outcome. Tables 1 and 2 show dietary data and cholesterol levels, respectively. Table 4 lists "other cardiovascular events." Note here that the largest differences (4.9% and 2.7%) are found in the two softest end points. The other end points listed under coronary disease have numbers too small to even merit consideration. The numbers for cerebrovascular events are likewise small but show no differences whatsoever. This is mildly interesting, because the types of symptoms and strokes included there are the closest thing from a pathophysiologic standpoint to MI; that is, they result from plaque disruption and blood clot formation in the arteries to the brain leading to strokes, just as the same process in the coronary arteries leads to heart attacks. In fact, these types of strokes are now often referred to as "brain attacks." Why cholesterol reduction should protect against this process in the heart but not the brain is never discussed.

Table 5 gives a summary of all the causes of death in both groups. This is a recurring burr under the saddle for the authors. It is interesting that they used the figures for combined definite *and suspected* CHD deaths (44 and 32) rather than those for only definite CHD deaths (38 and 30). This enabled them to increase the difference by 50% (from 8 to 12).

Had they used only the definite CHD death numbers, they would have a hard time explaining how that is significant when the cholestyramine group had seven more deaths due to accident or violence. Obviously, the increased deaths due to accidents and violence are mere happenstance and have nothing to do with taking cholesterol-lowering medication. If we apply the same statistical treatment to the differences in violent and accidental deaths, we could say that *not* taking cholestyramine reduced the risk of dying from these causes by 64% or, alternatively, that taking cholestyramine *caused* a 275% increase in deaths by accident or violence. These conclusions are absurd, but no more so than the authors' claim that taking cholestyramine reduced the risk of death from CHD by 24%.

The final section under the heading "Comment" is where the authors give their conclusions and their opinions on the implications of the results of their experiment. They begin with a flat statement that their trial "demonstrated that treatment with cholestyramine resin reduced the incidence of CHD." They then proceed to explain that they are sure that diet modification could accomplish the same result even though (they admit) no decent scientific study has ever shown that. They go on to say that other primary prevention studies failed to show a significant benefit to lowering cholesterol. They point out that some studies showed a lower incidence of fatal and nonfatal CHD but that "statistical significance was not attained." Of course, statistical significance was not attained in their study, either, until they changed the definition of significance to fit the outcome. (See *Commentary on the Published Results of the Lipid Research Clinics Coronary Primary Prevention Trial* by Dr. Richard A. Kronmal.)

Under the paragraph labeled "All-Cause Mortality," the authors again state that there was a 7% reduction in deaths from all causes in the treatment group. Once again, they give the figure for relative risk reduction rather than for absolute risk reduction (0.1%) and neglect to add that the difference was not statistically significant by anyone's criteria. The final sentence states that "Since no plausible connection could be established between cholestyramine treatment and violent or accidental death, it is difficult to conclude that this could be anything but a chance occurrence." This, of course, is certainly a true statement but could be equally well applied to the relationship between cholestyramine treatment and CHD death.

The final section, titled "Implications of the LRD-CPPT," reveals the authors' biases in their entirety. They say that although this trial wasn't designed to assess the value of diet, they feel that their findings "support the view that cholesterol lowering by diet also would be beneficial." This is purely a statement of their beliefs and is not justified by the findings in this or any other scientifically legitimate study. Although this claim is outrageous, they saved the best for last. After noting that the results could be narrowly interpreted as only applying to middle-aged men with very high cholesterol levels, they state that "the trial's implications, however, could and should be extended to other age groups and women and, since cholesterol levels and CHD risk are continuous variables to others with more modest elevations of cholesterol levels." Such an unwarranted extrapolation of their results is enough to remove any last shred of scientific credibility that may have attached to these authors.

The fine print at the conclusion of the paper tells us that the study was financed entirely by the National Heart, Lung, and Blood Institute (in other words, the taxpayers). There then follows a list of the locations of the twelve Lipid Research Clinics and a list of the principal investigators and key personnel in each. These days, all respectable medical journals require a potential conflict-of-interest disclosure statement from each of its authors showing their financial and other ties to drug companies or other businesses and organizations with a vested interest in the outcome of the study being presented. Fortunately, that wasn't customary at the time this article was published, or it would have added several more pages to the reprint.

# APPENDIX III

A. Original Report of the Helsinki Heart Study

B. How to Read and Interpret the Helsinki Heart Study Report.

# The New England
# Journal of Medicine

| Volume 317 | NOVEMBER 12, 1987 | Number 20 |

## HELSINKI HEART STUDY: PRIMARY-PREVENTION TRIAL WITH GEMFIBROZIL IN MIDDLE-AGED MEN WITH DYSLIPIDEMIA

### Safety of Treatment, Changes in Risk Factors, and Incidence of Coronary Heart Disease

M. Heikki Frick, M.D., Olli Elo, M.D., Kauko Haapa, M.D., Olli P. Heinonen, M.D., D.Sc.,
Pertti Heinsalmi, M.D., Pekka Helo, M.D., Jussi K. Huttunen, M.D., Pertti Kaitaniemi, M.D.,
Pekka Koskinen, M.D., Vesa Manninen, M.D., Hanna Mäenpää, M.D., Marjatta Mälkönen, M.Sc.,
Matti Mänttäri, M.D., Seppo Norola, M.D., Amos Pasternack, M.D., Jarmo Pikkarainen, M.D.,
Matti Romo, M.D., Tom Sjöblom, M.D., and Esko A. Nikkilä, M.D.*

**Abstract** In a randomized, double-blind five-year trial, we tested the efficacy of simultaneously elevating serum levels of high-density lipoprotein (HDL) cholesterol and lowering levels of non-HDL cholesterol with gemfibrozil in reducing the risk of coronary heart disease in 4081 asymptomatic middle-aged men (40 to 55 years of age) with primary dyslipidemia (non-HDL cholesterol ≥200 mg per deciliter [5.2 mmol per liter] in two consecutive pretreatment measurements). One group (2051 men) received 600 mg of gemfibrozil twice daily, and the other (2030 men) received placebo.

Gemfibrozil caused a marked increase in HDL cholesterol and persistent reductions in serum levels of total, low-density lipoprotein (LDL), and non-HDL cholesterol and triglycerides. There were minimal changes in serum lipid levels in the placebo group. The cumulative rate of cardiac end points at five years was 27.3 per 1000 in the gemfibrozil group and 41.4 per 1000 in the placebo group — a reduction of 34.0 percent in the incidence of coronary heart disease (95 percent confidence interval, 8.2 to 52.6; $P<0.02$; two-tailed test). The decline in incidence in the gemfibrozil group became evident in the second year and continued throughout the study. There was no difference between the groups in the total death rate, nor did the treatment influence the cancer rates.

The results are in accord with two previous trials with different pharmacologic agents and indicate that modification of lipoprotein levels with gemfibrozil reduces the incidence of coronary heart disease in men with dyslipidemia. (N Engl J Med 1987; 317:1237-45.)

A_N elevated serum level of low-density lipoprotein (LDL) cholesterol is a factor etiologically related to atherosclerotic vascular disease, and in particular to coronary heart disease.[1-5] A protective effect against coronary heart disease of elevated serum high-density lipoprotein (HDL) has been observed in several epidemiologic and clinical studies.[6-11] A low serum level of HDL cholesterol appears to be an important risk factor, particularly in populations whose serum level of total cholesterol is high.

Clinical trials aimed at reducing elevated serum total cholesterol (and hence LDL cholesterol) have demonstrated that whether the reduction is achieved by dietary or pharmacologic means, the incidence of coronary heart disease is reduced.[12-15] There is a positive correlation between the extent to which LDL choles-terol is lowered and the incidence of coronary heart disease.[16] No such conclusive data are so far available on the effect of induced changes in the serum level of HDL cholesterol on the incidence of coronary heart disease.

Gemfibrozil belongs to the group of fibric acid derivatives, but is structurally different and possesses biologic actions distinct from those of clofibrate.[17,18] Gemfibrozil reduces levels of total and LDL cholesterol and triglycerides, but also raises HDL cholesterol levels both in normal subjects and in patients with various forms of hyperlipoproteinemia.[19-28] The short-term toxicity of gemfibrozil is low, and no adverse effects due to long-term use have been reported.[20]

The Helsinki Heart Study was launched to investigate the effect of this agent on the incidence of coronary heart disease in a randomized, double-blind, five-year trial in middle-aged men who were free of coronary symptoms on entry and were at high risk because of abnormal concentrations of blood lipids.[29] The present report documents the changes in risk factors and the reduction in the incidence of coronary

From the First and Third Departments of Medicine, University of Helsinki; National Public Health Institute, Helsinki; Department of Medicine, University of Tampere, Finland; Finnish Railways, Posts and Telecommunications, and the following industrial companies: A. Ahlström, Enso-Gutzeit, Kaukas (Kymmene), Neste, and Veitsiluoto. Address reprint requests to Prof. Frick at the First Department of Medicine, University of Helsinki, SF-00290 Helsinki, Finland.

*Deceased, September 21, 1986.

heart disease, and provides an analysis of the major safety aspects of the trial.

## METHODS

### General Design

The design of the Helsinki Heart Study has been described in detail elsewhere.[30] The study was a randomized, double-blind, placebo-controlled trial of gemfibrozil (600 mg twice daily) against placebo, lasting for five years. In addition to drug treatment, a cholesterol-lowering diet was recommended to all participants. An increase in physical activity as well as a reduction in smoking and body weight was also encouraged.

The study protocol was approved by the Ethics Committee of the Faculty of Medicine, University of Helsinki; the National Board of Health in Finland; the U.S. Food and Drug Administration; and the trade unions and management of the public-sector and private-sector industries by whom the participants were employed. The study had a central office in Helsinki for its day-to-day management. There were 37 clinics, all of which followed the same protocol.

### Screening and Follow-up Procedures

On the basis of a pilot study,[30] non-HDL cholesterol, which is defined as total cholesterol minus HDL cholesterol (i.e., the sum of LDL and very-low-density lipoprotein [VLDL] cholesterol) was selected as the lipid whose level would determine acceptance into the study. Non-HDL cholesterol was considered to represent the atherogenic fractions in both the low-density and very-low-density regions of the lipoprotein distribution. The acceptance level was set at ≥200 mg per deciliter (5.2 mmol per liter). To ascertain that the lipid disorder was stable, the participant had to meet the acceptance criterion in two successive measurements.

The purpose of the screening was to identify at least 4000 healthy middle-aged men who satisfied the lipid acceptance criterion and were willing to participate in a five-year trial.[30] The participants were selected from 23,531 men 40 to 55 years of age who were employed by the Finnish Posts and Telecommunications agency, the Finnish State Railways, and five industrial companies in Finland. Complete screening of the civil service group was carried out during the first half of 1981, and the screening of the industrial employees one year later. A total of 18,966 men (80.6 percent) agreed to participate in the first screening. Subjects were excluded if they had any clinical manifestations of coronary heart disease or electrocardiographic abnormalities (713 men), congestive heart failure, or any other disease that could have had an influence on the study outcome. Subjects with hypertension and mild non-insulin-dependent diabetes were accepted.

The screening procedure was conducted in three steps and was completed in three to five months. During the first screening visit, blood pressure was measured and a blood sample with the subject not fasting was taken for the determination of serum levels of total and HDL cholesterol. Subjects fulfilling the lipid acceptance criterion and without reasons for exclusion (6903 men) were invited to the second screening visit, during which a medical examination was carried out and electrocardiography performed. A complete lipid profile in the fasting state and a multichannel laboratory analysis were obtained. At the third (base-line) visit, 4081 men who met the acceptance criterion and were willing to participate were randomly assigned to receive either gemfibrozil or placebo.

The subjects visited the clinics at three-month intervals. Data on compliance with the study regimen, adverse events, smoking, adherence to dietary recommendations, hospitalization, major illness, other medication, and any symptoms suggesting myocardial infarction were recorded, as were body weight and blood pressure. In any cases of suspected myocardial infarction, 12-lead electrocardiography was performed with the subject resting. In addition, routine electrocardiography was performed each year in conjunction with the annual medical examination.

Smoking habits were recorded in terms of the daily consumption of tobacco. Occupational and leisure-time physical activities were assessed with use of a four-point scale adapted from the Gothenburg study.[31] A modification of the Finnish version of the original Bortner rating scale for Type A behavior[32] was applied. Alcohol consumption was recorded according to the Scandinavian drinking survey.[33]

### Medication and Maintenance of Study Blinding

Subjects were randomly assigned to receive either gemfibrozil or placebo capsules in blocks distributed to each of the 37 clinics. The capsules were supplied by Parke–Davis Pharmaceutical Research Division, Pontypool, United Kingdom. Unused capsules were returned and counted. Gemfibrozil was measured in urine to check compliance, and the results were kept blinded for later analysis. A microdose of digoxin (2.2 μg per capsule) was used as a marker in both active and placebo capsules.[34] Urinary digoxin levels were measured in all participants during the last quarter of the third[35] and fifth study years.

Every effort was made to maintain the double-blindness of the study. A four-member safety committee had access to safety data. The committee reviewed the end points of the study according to treatment group only once during the trial. The end points, along with the codes, were sealed and kept in a safe until all patients had completed the trial.

### Laboratory Methods

A venous blood sample was drawn into a vacuum tube at every visit. A sample in the fasting state was required during the semiannual visits only, when the serum concentration of triglycerides was determined. Serum samples were sent to the central laboratory (at the National Public Health Institute in Helsinki) daily by mail. The interval from sampling to analysis ranged from one to five days. The total cholesterol was measured directly in the serum, and HDL cholesterol was measured after precipitation of VLDL and LDL with dextran sulfate–magnesium chloride by an enzymatic method.[30] The concentration of triglycerides in serum was determined by measuring glycerol after an enzymatic hydrolysis with lipase–esterase.[30] The LDL cholesterol concentration was calculated according to the formula LDL cholesterol = total cholesterol minus HDL cholesterol minus triglycerides divided by 5.[36]

The mean coefficients of variation from day to day for total cholesterol and HDL cholesterol were 0.9 percent and 2.0 percent, respectively. External quality assessments were made in collaboration with the World Health Organization Lipid Research Center in Prague. The mean deviation from reference values was ±0.5 percent, and the range was −1.5 to 1.0 percent for the total cholesterol level. The accuracy of the cholesterol method was further tested against quality-control serum samples analyzed by mass spectrometry. The deviation from the reference cholesterol value was ±0.4 percent.

Because the triglyceride concentration was not measured at the base-line visit (the last before treatment), the base-line values for LDL cholesterol were calculated on the basis of total cholesterol and HDL cholesterol values at the base-line visit and triglyceride values determined at the second screening visit. Triglyceride values of 700 mg per deciliter or higher were excluded from the LDL calculations.[36] LDL cholesterol values under 100 mg per deciliter (e.g., negative values) were deemed outliers and were excluded.

In addition to hemoglobin measurements, white-cell counts, and strip tests for urinary sugar and protein performed in local laboratories twice a year, a package analysis was carried out in the central laboratory to measure the following: alkaline phosphatase, aspartate aminotransferase, bilirubin, calcium, creatinine, iron, latent iron-binding capacity, and uric acid.

### Cardiovascular End Points

Fatal and nonfatal myocardial infarction and cardiac death were the principal end points. All end-point assessments were made without knowledge of the subject's treatment. Classifications could not be altered once the treatment codes were broken. "Fatal myocardial infarction" was diagnosed when a death certificate or hospital record described the cause of death and there was either preterminal hospitalization with definite myocardial infarction or an autopsy finding of acute myocardial infarction. "Sudden cardiac death" was diagnosed when a death certificate described coronary heart disease and death occurred within one hour after the onset of symptoms.

Vol. 317   No. 20       GEMFIBROZIL AND CORONARY HEART DISEASE — FRICK ET AL.       1239

"Unwitnessed cardiac death" was diagnosed when a death certificate described coronary heart disease and there was no evidence to justify a classification of sudden cardiac death.

"Definite nonfatal myocardial infarction" was diagnosed in hospitalized patients when there was a diagnostic electrocardiogram at the time of the event (Minnesota codes[37] 1-1, or 1-2 plus 5-1 or 5-2, and excluding 1-2.6 and 1-2.8) or ischemic cardiac pain and diagnostic enzyme levels (levels of aspartate aminotransferase, creatine kinase, creatine kinase MB, or lactate dehydrogenase exceeding at least twice the upper limit of the reference values) or ischemic cardiac pain and equivocal enzyme levels (elevated but not fulfilling the diagnostic criteria) and an equivocal electrocardiogram (Minnesota codes 1-2 or 1-3, 4-I-1 to 4-I-3, 5-1 to 5-2, or 7-1). In patients not hospitalized, the diagnosis was confirmed when a patient reporting chest pain, breathlessness, or syncope had a diagnostic electrocardiogram at the time of the event or when annual routine electrocardiography indicated new changes consistent with myocardial infarction.

Hospitalized patients with ischemic cardiac pain and equivocal enzyme levels or an equivocal electrocardiogram were classified as having a "possible myocardial infarction," whereas among patients not hospitalized, ischemic cardiac pain and an electrocardiogram that was equivocal for reasons other than S-T-segment or T-wave changes were sufficient criteria. Possible myocardial infarction was not considered a cardiovascular end point. The classification of definite and possible cases was made by a senior board-certified cardiologist. A more detailed description of the end-point definitions has been published.[30]

The Minnesota coding of the electrocardiograms was performed by two specially trained technicians. All positive findings were checked by an independent board-certified cardiologist, who also had no clinical information about the participants. To check the reliability of negative findings, a review committee, consisting of two independent cardiologists with experience in cardiovascular epidemiology and clinical cardiology, reviewed a random sample of Minnesota codings. A board-certified cardiologist who was a member of the research group made the end-point assessment, using the Minnesota coding and all relevant clinical information, including data on enzymes.

The review committee evaluated the classification of all end points. In the few cases in which there was a difference of opinion between the designated cardiologist and the review committee, the final assessment of an end point was made by the four-member safety committee, consisting of experts in clinical cardiology and cardiovascular epidemiology.

### Statistical Methods

The log-rank (Mantel–Haenszel) statistic[38] was used to compare the survival (or failure) curves in the treatment groups. The nominal P value derived by this procedure is reported, as well as the corresponding two-tailed 5 percent critical chi-square value derived by the sequential procedure of Lan and DeMets.[39] This procedure has been recommended for the analysis of survival-type data in long-term clinical trials.[40] In determining the Lan–DeMets critical value, time in the study was approximated by calendar time. Thus, the one interim analysis occurred in 71.4 percent of the way through the study. The 5 percent alpha-error rate was "spent" with use of the function $\alpha * (t)$, to approximate the O'Brien–Fleming boundaries.[41] The Kaplan–Meier method was used to construct life-table plots.[42]

### RESULTS

#### Success of Random Assignment

A total of 18,966 subjects were screened, and 4081 were included in the trial (Table 1). They were randomly assigned to receive either gemfibrozil (2051 men) or placebo (2030 men). With the exception of serum lipids, the levels of other cardiovascular risk factors were almost identical in the screened population and in the two treatment groups. Because the first screening was not carried out in the fasting state, tri-

Table 1. Characteristics of the Screened Population and the Treatment Groups at the First Screening in the Helsinki Heart Study.*

| CHARACTERISTIC | SCREENED POPULATION | TREATMENT GROUP | |
| --- | --- | --- | --- |
| | | GEMFIBROZIL | PLACEBO |
| No. of subjects | 18,966 | 2051 | 2030 |
| | | mean ±SD | |
| Age (yr) | 47.3±4.7 | 47.2±4.6 | 47.4±4.6 |
| Body-mass index (kg/m²) | 26.3±3.2 | 26.6±3.2 | 26.6±3.2 |
| Blood pressure (mm Hg) | | | |
| Systolic | 141.0±17.1 | 142.1±16.6 | 141.3±16.4 |
| Diastolic | 90.3±10.5 | 91.5±10.2 | 91.0±10.2 |
| Cholesterol (mg/dl)† | | | |
| Total | 244.7±45.1 | 289.1±32.9 | 288.7±31.3 |
| HDL | 49.4±11.9 | 47.1±10.5 | 47.1±11.0 |
| Non-HDL‡ | 195.4±45.9 | 242.1±32.2 | 241.7±30.8 |
| Triglycerides (mg/dl)§ | ND | 175.3±117.8 | 176.6±120.5 |
| | | percent of total | |
| Hypertension¶ | 12.9 | 14.5 | 13.4 |
| Diabetes | 2.6 | 2.4 | 2.9 |
| Nonsmokers | 40.2 | 37.2 | 35.7 |
| Exsmokers | 27.5 | 26.4 | 28.5 |
| Smokers | 32.3 | 36.5 | 35.8 |
| Fredrickson type | | | |
| IIa | ND | 63.3 | 63.7 |
| IIb | ND | 27.9 | 27.5 |
| IV | ND | 8.8 | 8.5 |

*HDL denotes high-density lipoprotein, and ND not determined in the first screening.
†To convert values to millimoles per liter, multiply by 0.02586.
‡Total cholesterol minus HDL cholesterol.
§To convert values to millimoles per liter, multiply by 0.01129.
¶Hypertension was defined as one screening blood pressure of >170/≥100 mm Hg, or a diastolic pressure >105 mm Hg; it was also considered present if the patient was taking antihypertensive medication.

glyceride values were available for only 6903 subjects who participated in the second screening — i.e., whose non-HDL cholesterol level was ≥200 mg per deciliter (5.2 mmol per liter) at the first screening. Their mean serum triglyceride level was 171.7 mg per deciliter (1.94 mmol per liter) — slightly below the value in the two treatment groups.

The mean blood pressure, the rate of smoking, and the prevalence of hypertension, diabetes, and the customary Fredrickson lipoprotein types IIa, IIb, and IV were similar in the two treatment groups (Table 1). The gemfibrozil and placebo groups were also similar with regard to their scores on the Bortner behavior-rating scale, alcohol consumption, and family history of myocardial infarction and angina pectoris.[30] The leisure-time physical-activity score was significantly higher in the placebo than in the gemfibrozil group. Finally, the predicted five-year incidences of coronary heart disease according to the multiple logistic risk functions were similar in both treatment groups, as they were when analyzed in subgroups of occupational affiliation and geographic area.[30]

#### Study Participation and Compliance with Medication Regimen

Of the total 4081 subjects initially randomized, 2859 (70.1 percent) continued in the trial until its completion. In the gemfibrozil group, the annual dropout rates among subjects remaining in the study from the previous year were 14.7, 6.6, 5.3, 4.7, and 4.5 percent, respectively. In the placebo group, the rates were 12.6, 6.4, 4.5, 4.3, and 4.4 percent. All the subjects initially randomized were followed for five years and included in the analysis; none were lost to follow-up.

According to the three-month capsule counts, the proportions of prescribed capsules taken annually in the gemfibrozil group were 85, 85, 84, 84, and 82 percent. The respective figures for the placebo group were 85, 86, 86, 86, and 83 percent. The digoxin-marker study also indicated that the compliance with the regimen was good.[35]

### Blood Lipids

The last of the three pretreatment lipid values, measured when the drug or placebo was dispensed, was chosen to represent the base-line value for the subsequent follow-up, since there was a declining trend during the screening period, except for HDL, which did not change. Before the intervention, triglycerides were measured only during the second screening.

During treatment, the placebo group had only minimal and random changes from the base-line values and particularly clear seasonal variations. Gemfibrozil rapidly increased the HDL cholesterol level by more than 10 percent; this was followed by a small decline with time. The total cholesterol level was initially reduced by 11 percent, the level of LDL cholesterol by 10 percent, that of non-HDL cholesterol by 14 percent, and that of triglycerides by 43 percent; these changes were followed by a consistent level of total and of LDL cholesterol and a small increase in the triglyceride level during the last years of the trial (Fig. 1; Table 2). These changes resulted in significant and sustained elevations in the ratios of HDL cholesterol to LDL cholesterol and of HDL cholesterol to total cholesterol.

### Selected Cardiovascular Risk Factors

Systolic and diastolic blood pressure, body mass, and smoking habits remained similar in both treatment groups throughout the study. Changes in blood pressure were within 1 mm Hg, changes in body-mass index were within 0.2 kg per square meter, and smoking decreased 3 to 4 percent in both treatment groups.

### Cardiac End Points

The mean follow-up period was 60.4 months, and the total follow-up period was 20,541 person-years. The total dropout rate was 29.9 percent. If the dropouts are taken into account, the total exposure to gemfibrozil was 8194 person-years, as opposed to 8372 person-years for the placebo.

The total number of cardiac end points in the gemfibrozil group was 56 (27.3 per 1000), as compared with 84 in the placebo group (41.4 per 1000) (Table

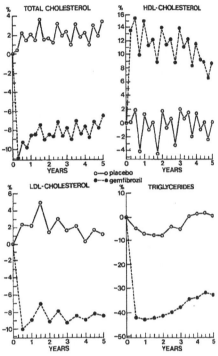

Figure 1. Percentage Changes in Lipid Values from Base Line, According to Treatment Group and Time.

3), yielding a log-rank chi-square of 6.0, with a nominal $P<0.02$ (two-tailed). The significance was also tested according to the Lan–DeMets procedure, taking into account the interim evaluation of the data at three years. With this conservative procedure, the difference between the two groups was also statistically significant (critical value = 4.02; $P<0.05$; two-tailed). The overall reduction in the frequency of cardiac end points in the gemfibrozil group was 34.0 percent (95 percent confidence interval, 8.2 to 52.6).

The greatest reduction in end-point rates (37 percent; $P<0.05$) was noted in the group with nonfatal myocardial infarction (21.9 per 1000 vs. 35.0 per 1000; $P<0.02$). The results were essentially similar when the analysis excluded the patients who dropped out. The end-point rates in the civil service group were 25.2 per 1000 for gemfibrozil and 44.3 per 1000 for placebo. The respective values in the industrial group were 31.3 per 1000 and 35.9 per 1000. The distribution of end points from clinic to clinic favored gemfibrozil in 29 of the 37 centers in the study; most of the remaining centers showed equal distributions of the end points.

The Kaplan–Meier life-table values for the cumula-

Vol. 317   No. 20          GEMFIBROZIL AND CORONARY HEART DISEASE — FRICK ET AL.          1241

Table 2. Lipid Values According to Treatment Group and Time.*

| SERUM LIPID | | GEMFIBROZIL | | | PLACEBO | | |
|---|---|---|---|---|---|---|---|
| Interval (mo) ⟶ | | BASE LINE | 0–24 | ≥25 | BASE LINE | 0–24 | ≥25 |
| Cholesterol (mg/dl) | | | | | | | |
| Total | Mean | 269.9 | 244.7 | 246.9 | 269.6 | 272.5 | 272.6 |
| | SE | 0.78 | 0.76 | 0.85 | 0.78 | 0.71 | 0.78 |
| | No. | 2051 | 1973 | 1611 | 2030 | 1958 | 1638 |
| HDL | Mean | 47.1 | 52.1 | 51.2 | 47.6 | 46.8 | 47.0 |
| | SE | 0.24 | 0.26 | 0.29 | 0.25 | 0.23 | 0.26 |
| | No. | 2051 | 1973 | 1611 | 2030 | 1958 | 1638 |
| Non-HDL† | Mean | 222.9 | 192.6 | 195.7 | 222.1 | 225.7 | 225.5 |
| | SE | 0.78 | 0.80 | 0.89 | 0.78 | 0.72 | 0.78 |
| | No. | 2051 | 1973 | 1611 | 2030 | 1958 | 1638 |
| LDL | Mean | 189.2 | 172.8 | 173.5 | 188.2 | 193.6 | 191.4 |
| | SE | 0.76 | 0.72 | 0.77 | 0.76 | 0.70 | 0.76 |
| | No. | 2004 | 1885 | 1590 | 1991 | 1887 | 1616 |
| Cholesterol ratio | | | | | | | |
| HDL to total | Mean | 0.18 | 0.22 | 0.21 | 0.18 | 0.17 | 0.17 |
| | SE | 0.00 | 0.00 | 0.00 | 0.00 | 0.00 | 0.00 |
| | No. | 2051 | 1973 | 1611 | 2030 | 1958 | 1638 |
| HDL to LDL | Mean | 0.26 | 0.32 | 0.31 | 0.26 | 0.25 | 0.26 |
| | SE | 0.00 | 0.00 | 0.00 | 0.00 | 0.00 | 0.00 |
| | No. | 2004 | 1885 | 1590 | 1991 | 1887 | 1616 |
| Triglycerides (mg/dl)‡ | Mean | 175.3 | 102.7 | 114.8 | 176.7 | 166.6 | 177.7 |
| | SE | 2.60 | 1.38 | 1.68 | 2.67 | 2.10 | 2.34 |
| | No. | 2050 | 1885 | 1590 | 2030 | 1891 | 1618 |

*Values are means of readings made during the indicated intervals. HDL denotes high-density lipoprotein, and LDL low-density lipoprotein. To convert cholesterol values to millimoles per liter, multiply by 0.02586. To convert triglyceride values to millimoles per liter, multiply by 0.01129.

†Total cholesterol minus HDL cholesterol.

‡Not determined at base line. Values shown were obtained at the second screening.

tive incidence of definite cardiac end points, as well as the actual annual number of definite end points, are shown in Figure 2. No meaningful difference was observed during the first two years. Thereafter, the curves began to separate, with a progressive decrease in the gemfibrozil group, whereas the annual end-point rate in the placebo group remained virtually unaltered throughout the study. From the third to fifth years of the trial, the number of end points in the gemfibrozil group was about one-third to one-half their number in the placebo group. In the fifth year, there were 6 end points in the gemfibrozil group and 18 in the placebo group when analysis was performed on an intention-to-treat basis. If the dropouts were excluded, the corresponding numbers of end points were 4 and 16, respectively.

There were 31 cases of possible myocardial infarction (15 in the gemfibrozil group and 16 in the placebo group). When these cases were included in the analyses, the difference in end-point rates between treatment groups was still statistically significant.

### Mortality

There were 45 deaths (rate, 21.9 per 1000) in the gemfibrozil group and 42 deaths (rate, 20.7 per 1000) in the placebo group (Table 4). This difference was not statistically significant. Neither were there significant differences between the treatment groups in any of the specific causes of death. There were fewer deaths due to ischemic heart disease and more deaths due to violence, accidents, and intracranial hemorrhage in the gemfibrozil group, but the dif-

ferences were not statistically significant.

### Cancers

There was no significant difference in the total number of cancers (31 vs. 26) between the two treatment groups (Table 5). In the subgroup analysis, there were five basal-cell carcinomas of the skin in the gemfibrozil group and none in the placebo group. This difference was of borderline statistical significance according to Fisher's exact test (P = 0.062). The expected numbers of basal-cell carcinomas calculated from the national cancer statistics of Finland[43] were 4.8 cases in the gemfibrozil group and 4.7 in the placebo group. No statistically significant differences were found in any of the analyses of other specific cancer types.

### Surgical Operations and Hospital Admissions

In the subgroup analyses according to type of operation, there were no significant differences between the treatment groups in the numbers of any major surgical operations. In particular, gemfibrozil did not significantly increase the number of gallstone operations (18 in the gemfibrozil group vs. 12 in the placebo group). However, when all gastrointestinal operations, including hemorrhoidectomies, were combined, there was a statistically significant difference (81 in the gemfibrozil group vs. 53 in the placebo group, P<0.02). Eye operations were somewhat more common in the gemfibrozil group (17 vs. 12), mainly because of cataract operations (7 vs. 3), but the differences were not statistically significant. The same applied to coronary-bypass surgery (7 vs. 6).

When hospital admissions for the treatment of acute myocardial infarction were excluded, there were no statistically significant differences between the two treatment groups in the total numbers of hospitalizations or in the numbers of hospitalizations for gastrointestinal diseases or symptoms.

### Adverse Events

During the first year, 11.3 percent of the subjects in the gemfibrozil group reported various moderate to severe upper gastrointestinal symptoms, whereas the corresponding rate for the placebo group was 7.0 percent (P<0.001). During subsequent years, these rates decreased to 2.4 and 1.2 percent (P<0.05), respectively. No significant differences between treatment groups were observed in the occurrence of constipation, diarrhea, or nausea and vomiting.

Similarly, no differences between the two treatment

Table 3. Cardiac End Points and Cases of Possible Myocardial Infarction According to Treatment Group and Participation Status.

| CORONARY EVENT | SUBJECTS RECEIVING TREATMENT | | SUBJECTS WITHDRAWN FROM TREATMENT | | TOTAL | |
|---|---|---|---|---|---|---|
| | GEMFIBROZIL | PLACEBO | GEMFIBROZIL | PLACEBO | GEMFIBROZIL | PLACEBO |
| | | | | | no. (rate/1000) | |
| Definite | | | | | | |
| Nonfatal myocardial infarction | 40 | 61 | 5 | 10 | 45 (21.9) | 71 (35.0) |
| Fatal myocardial infarction | 3 | 7 | 3 | 1 | 6 (2.9) | 8 (3.9) |
| Sudden cardiac death | 3 | 3 | 2 | 1 | 5 (2.4) | 4 (2.0) |
| Unwitnessed death | 0 | 1 | 0 | 0 | 0 (0.0) | 1 (0.5) |
| Total | 46 | 72 | 10 | 12 | 56 (27.3) | 84 (41.4)* |
| Possible | 14 | 12 | 1 | 4 | 15 (7.3) | 16 (7.9) |

*Log-rank chi-square = 6.0; nominal P value <0.02 (two-tailed). Lan–DeMets sequential-procedure critical value = 4.02; overall P value <0.05 (two-tailed).

groups were observed in levels of hemoglobin, urinary protein, or urinary sugar or in laboratory multichannel analyses.

## DISCUSSION

The total rate of cardiac end points during the five-year study was 27.3 per 1000 in the gemfibrozil group and 41.4 per 1000 in the placebo group (log-rank P<0.02, two-tailed). The number of definite cardiac end points was 56 in the gemfibrozil group and 84 in the placebo group. Despite a 26 percent lower mortality from coronary heart disease (19 vs. 14), there were slightly more deaths overall in the gemfibrozil

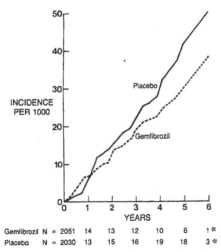

Gemfibrozil N = 2051    14    13    12    10    6    1 ☆
Placebo    N = 2030    13    15    16    19    18    3 ☆

Figure 2. Kaplan–Meier Cumulative Incidence (per 1000) and Annual Number of Cardiac End Points, According to Treatment Group and Time.

Data for the sixth year (stars) were derived from 305 person-years of observation for gemfibrozil and from 316 person-years of observation for placebo.

than in the placebo group (45 vs. 42). The size of the study population and the length of observation were not, however, sufficient to allow conclusions about the possible effects of changes in cardiac mortality on total mortality. The higher number of deaths in the gemfibrozil group was mainly due to accidents or violence and intracranial hemorrhage. An excess number of violent deaths in subjects treated with lipid-lowering regimens has also been observed in other studies[44] but has been interpreted to be a chance finding. No significant difference was observed between the groups in the occurrence of neoplasms.

A 30 percent reduction in the incidence of coronary heart disease was considered during the planning stage of the study to be the minimal change necessary to justify the use of long-term medication in subjects without symptoms. The observed reduction was 34 percent over the entire study period and more than 50 percent during years three to five. The difference during the latter half of the study may represent the long-term effect of the drug, since earlier studies[14,44] also suggest a lag of one to three years between the start of lipid-lowering treatment and effects on morbidity from coronary heart disease. A latent period between the changes in lipid values and changes in morbidity has also been predicted on the basis of epidemiologic studies[45] and may in fact be expected, because of the slow progress of the underlying atherosclerotic process.[46,47]

The incidence of events related to coronary heart disease in the placebo group was lower than expected — 41 per 1000 as compared with a predicted rate of 75 per 1000 in five years. Estimates of the incidence of coronary heart disease in men with similar dyslipidemia were based on coronary-register data collected in the 1970s.[30] This lower-than-predicted rate has also been observed in several previous clinical trials and may be due to a number of factors, including stringent selection processes, better health monitoring, and the concurrent decline in mortality and morbidity from coronary heart disease in the general population.

Previous dietary and pharmacologic trials have attempted to show that modification of lipid levels results in decreased morbidity and mortality from coronary heart disease. A statistically significant reduction was observed in patients on a fat-modified diet in the Finnish mental hospital study[12] and in conjunction with an antismoking program in the Oslo study.[13] Earlier pharmacologic trials, such as the World Health Organization's study of clofibrate[14] and the Lipid Research Clinic's (LRC) Coronary Primary Prevention Trial of cholestyramine[14] have both demonstrated that lowering cholesterol levels with drugs

Vol. 317   No. 20        GEMFIBROZIL AND CORONARY HEART DISEASE — FRICK ET AL.        1243

Table 4. Deaths According to Treatment Group and Cause.*

| CAUSE OF DEATH | GEMFIBROZIL | | PLACEBO | |
|---|---|---|---|---|
| | NO. | RATE/1000 | NO. | RATE/1000 |
| Ischemic heart disease | 14† | 6.8 | 19‡ | 9.4 |
| Ischemic cerebral infarction | 1 | 0.5 | 3 | 1.5 |
| Intracranial hemorrhage | 5§ | 2.4 | 1 | 0.5 |
| Other vascular cause | 2 | 1.0 | 0 | 0.0 |
| Malignant neoplasm | 11 | 5.4 | 11 | 5.4 |
| Other medical cause | 2 | 1.0 | 4 | 2.0 |
| Accident/violence | 10 | 4.9 | 4 | 2.0 |
| Total | 45 | 21.9 | 42 | 20.7 |

*The differences in rates between the treatment groups were not statistically significant.
†Three subjects died later in the study after surviving initial myocardial infarction.
‡Six subjects died later in the study after surviving initial myocardial infarction.
§One subject had pulmonary embolism and hemorrhage after streptokinase treatment.

significantly decreases the incidence of major coronary events. In the World Health Organization study there was, however, an increase in mortality due to a variety of causes, with no particular disease predominating. This excess of deaths diverted attention from the principal study finding — i.e., that reduction of plasma cholesterol lowered the incidence of coronary heart disease.

The LRC cholestyramine study was a multicenter, randomized, double-blind investigation to test the efficacy of cholesterol lowering in reducing the risk of coronary heart disease in 3806 asymptomatic men with hypercholesterolemia that had not responded to simple dietary management.[15,44] In many respects, the LRC trial and the Helsinki heart study are similar. In both studies, the participants (in the LRC study, men 35 to 59 years of age; in the Helsinki study, men 40 to 55) were initially free of overt coronary heart disease and other major disabilities. The LRC study had as its initial entry criteria a total cholesterol level over 265 mg per deciliter (6.85 mmol per liter) and an LDL cholesterol level over 175 mg per deciliter (4.53 mmol per liter) after a period of dietary intervention. Subjects were excluded if they had serum triglyceride levels over 300 mg per deciliter (3.4 mmol per liter), hypertension, or some other diseases.

Table 5. Cancers According to Treatment Group.*

| CANCER | GEMFIBROZIL | | PLACEBO | |
|---|---|---|---|---|
| | NO. | RATE/1000 | NO. | RATE/1000 |
| Lung | 5 | 2.4 | 5 | 2.5 |
| Colon/rectum | 3 | 1.5 | 4 | 2.0 |
| Stomach | 1 | 0.5 | 4 | 2.0 |
| Leukemia | 2 | 1.0 | 1 | 0.5 |
| Skin: basal-cell carcinoma | 5 | 2.4 | 0 | 0.0 |
| Other | 15† | — | 12‡ | — |
| Total | 31 | 15.1 | 26 | 12.8 |

*The differences in rates between treatment groups were not statistically significant, except for the differences in basal-cell carcinoma (P = 0.032 by Fisher's exact test).

†Cancers of the brain, bladder, bile duct, esophagus, gall bladder, liver, nasopharynx, prostate, kidney, and thyroid, and femoral fibrosarcoma, glioblastoma, lymphoma, melanoma, and myeloma.

‡Anaplastic cancer, carcinoid tumor of the small intestine, fibrosarcoma, intestinal mesothelioma, myeloma (two cases), pancreatic cancer (two), peritoneal fibrosarcoma, renal cancer (two), and type not specified (one).

Thus, all the patients in the LRC trial had Type II hyperlipoproteinemia.

Both the initial and final criterion of the Helsinki heart study was a level of non-HDL cholesterol equal to or greater than 200 mg per deciliter (5.2 mmol per liter). This criterion yielded 9 percent patients with Type IV hyperlipoproteinemia, 28 percent with Type IIb, and 63 percent with Type IIa. In spite of these differences, the initial mean lipid values were almost identical in the two studies. On the other hand, the two drugs used have distinctly different effects and mechanisms of action. Cholestyramine, a nonabsorbable sequestrant of bile acid, effectively lowers LDL cholesterol but has only minimal effects on VLDL and HDL cholesterol. In contrast, gemfibrozil elevates HDL cholesterol and reduces LDL and VLDL cholesterol.[17-28]

The cholestyramine-treated subjects in the seven-year LRC study had average reductions in plasma levels of total and LDL cholesterol of 13 and 20 percent, respectively, and an average increase in HDL cholesterol of 3 percent. A 21 percent reduction (38 vs. 30) in definite coronary deaths and a 17 percent reduction (187 vs. 155) in all definite end points for coronary heart disease were observed. Treatment with gemfibrozil in the Helsinki heart study over the five-year period induced mean reductions in serum total cholesterol, LDL cholesterol, non-HDL cholesterol, and triglycerides, respectively, of 8, 8, 12, and 35 percent, and an increase of more than 10 percent in HDL cholesterol. All lipid responses in the Helsinki heart study were obvious three to six months after the start of drug treatment. The differences between the gemfibrozil and placebo groups were maintained throughout the five-year study. These changes were accompanied by a 26 percent reduction in definite coronary deaths (19 vs. 14) and a 34 percent reduction in all definite end points for coronary heart disease (84 vs. 56).

It is generally agreed that ideal total cholesterol values should be below 200 mg per deciliter (5.2 mmol per liter)[48,49] and that active treatment should certainly be instituted in subjects with values in excess of 250 mg per deciliter (6.5 mmol per liter). On the other hand, no such definite guidelines have been generated for levels of HDL cholesterol. The study group of the European Atherosclerosis Society provisionally set a cutoff point of 35 mg per deciliter for the lower limit of plasma HDL cholesterol.[48] Several sources indicate that levels of HDL cholesterol should be at least 20 percent of total cholesterol in populations with high levels of non-HDL cholesterol.[7,10,11] In view of the growing evidence of the protective role of HDL in atherogenesis,[6-11] it is logical to raise the level of this lipoprotein either by nonpharmacologic means (exercise and weight reduction) or by pharmacologic means, at least in persons with high levels of non-HDL cholesterol. The present results are in agreement with such an approach. A simultaneous increase in HDL cholesterol and reduction in non-HDL choles-

1244    THE NEW ENGLAND JOURNAL OF MEDICINE    Nov. 12, 1987

terol with gemfibrozil significantly reduced the incidence of coronary heart disease in middle-aged men.

The greatest relative change in serum lipid levels (approximately 35 percent) that was observed in this study was that in serum triglycerides. The role of triglycerides as a coronary risk factor is still controversial. The existing information suggests that in the presence of normal cholesterol levels, small elevations of plasma triglyceride levels do not necessarily increase the risk of cardiovascular disease. However, triglyceride levels exceeding 250 mg per deciliter (2.8 mmol per liter) may be associated with an increased risk of coronary heart disease, particularly in young subjects.[50-52] Whether the association is causal and the treatment of hypertriglyceridemia, either by dietary or pharmacologic means, is justified remains to be established.

The cancer mortality was identical in the two treatment groups. The small excess in the incidence of basal-cell carcinomas in the gemfibrozil group will require further evaluation, since the rate in the placebo group was exceptionally low.[43] The incidence of other neoplasms did not differ between the study groups.

The use of gemfibrozil resulted in several gastrointestinal side effects, although these were also common in the placebo group. Although according to one study gemfibrozil is less lithogenic than clofibrate,[18] it increases biliary cholesterol saturation in healthy persons,[53] and this may cause more gallstones and necessitate more cholecystectomies. There were slightly more cases of eye surgery, mainly involving cataracts, in the gemfibrozil than in the placebo group. None of the differences between the two study groups in the numbers of surgical operations for specific causes were statistically significant.

In conclusion, specifically modifying the lipoprotein profile with gemfibrozil resulted in a marked reduction in the incidence of coronary heart disease without evoking any critical adverse events. These findings are in accord with those of two previous primary-prevention trials using lipid-modulating agents with different pharmacologic effects,[14,15,44] and furnish additional and conclusive evidence of the role of lipid modification in preventing coronary heart disease.

We are indebted to the participants in the study for their understanding and trust; to the nurses for their excellent care; to Stephen Preston, M.D., John Gorringe, M.D., Robert Hodges, M.D., and Mr. Joseph Dresner for overseeing the initial phases of the study and for subsequent help; to David Evans, M.D., and Mr. Roy Couch for extremely valuable contributions; to Terry Goodburn, Ph.D., and his department in Pontypool, United Kingdom, who supplied the drugs; to Ms. Kaija Javela and her staff for excellent work at the Central Laboratory of the Public Health Institute; to Sven Punsar, M.D., Ritva Halonen, R.N., and Outi Marila, R.N., for the excellent quality of the electrocardiogram reading and the Minnesota coding; to Pentti Ristola, M.D., and Olli Suhonen, M.D., who liberally gave their time and expertise for the independent end-point revision; to Mr. Joe Dresner (director), Mr. Harry Haber, Ms. Janet Ward, and the whole staff of the data-processing section in Ann Arbor, Michigan, for excellent service in managing well over half a million case reports and other information collected during the study; and to the Warner–Lambert Company and all the Finnish participating institutions for their generous support.

Tables concerning selected risk factors and their changes during the study, as well as surgical operations and gastrointestinal side effects, can be obtained on request from the authors.

## REFERENCES

1. Keys A. Seven countries: a multivariate analysis of death and coronary heart disease. Cambridge, Mass.: Harvard University Press, 1980.
2. Dawber TR. The Framingham Study: the epidemiology of atherosclerotic disease. Cambridge, Mass.: Harvard University Press, 1980.
3. American Heart Association Steering Committee for Medical and Community Program. Risk factors and coronary disease: a statement for physicians. Circulation 1980; 62:449A-455A.
4. Ross R. The pathology of atherosclerosis — an update. N Engl J Med 1986; 314:488-500.
5. Martin MJ, Hulley SB, Browner WS, Kuller LH, Wentworth D. Serum cholesterol, blood pressure, and mortality: implications from a cohort of 361 662 men. Lancet 1986; 2:933-6.
6. Barr DP, Russ EM, Eder HA. Protein-lipid relationships in human plasma. II. In atherosclerosis and related conditions. Am J Med 1951; 11:480-93.
7. Nikkilä E. Studies on the lipid-protein relationships in normal and pathological sera and the effect of heparin on serum lipoproteins. Scand J Clin Lab Invest [Suppl] 1953; 5:Suppl 8:1-101.
8. Miller GJ, Miller NE. Plasma-high-density-lipoprotein concentration and development of ischaemic heart-disease. Lancet 1975; 1:16-9.
9. Miller NE, Førde OH, Thelle DS, Mjøs OD. The Tromsø Heart-Study: high-density lipoprotein and coronary heart-disease: a prospective case-control study. Lancet 1977; 1:965-7.
10. Gordon T, Castelli WP, Hjortland MC, Kannel WB, Dawber TR. High density lipoprotein as a protective factor against coronary heart disease. Am J Med 1977; 62:707-14.
11. Castelli WP, Garrison RJ, Wilson PWF, Abbott RD, Kalousdian S, Kannel WB. Incidence of coronary heart disease and lipoprotein cholesterol levels: the Framingham Study. JAMA 1986; 256:2835-8.
12. Turpeinen O, Karvonen MJ, Pekkarinen M, Miettinen M, Elosuo R, Paavilainen E. Dietary prevention of coronary heart disease: the Finnish Mental Hospital Study. Int J Epidemiol 1979; 8:99-118.
13. Hjermann I, Velve Byre K, Holme I, Leren P. Effect of diet and smoking intervention on the incidence of coronary heart disease: report from the Oslo Study Group of a randomized trial in healthy men. Lancet 1981; 2:1303-10.
14. Oliver MF, Heady JA, Morris JN, et al. A co-operative trial in the primary prevention of ischaemic heart disease using clofibrate: a report from the Committee of Principal Investigators. Br Heart J 1978; 40:1069-118.
15. Lipid Research Clinics Program. The Lipid Research Clinics Coronary Primary Prevention Trial results. II. The relationship of reduction in incidence of coronary heart disease to cholesterol lowering. JAMA 1984; 251:365-74.
16. Peto R, Yusuf S, Collins R. Cholesterol-lowering trial results in their epidemiologic context. Circulation 1985; 72:III-451. abstract.
17. Gemfibrozil: a new lipid lowering agent: proceedings of an International Symposium held by Parke, Davis & Company at The Royal Society of Medicine on 15–16 June 1976. Proc R Soc Med 1976; 69:Suppl 2:1-120.
18. Newton RS, Krause BR. Mechanisms of action of gemfibrozil: comparison of studies in the rat to clinical efficacy: In: Fears R, ed. Pharmacological control of hyperlipidaemia. Barcelona, Spain: J.R. Prous, 1986: 171-86.
19. Nikkilä EA, Ylikahri R, Huttunen JK. Gemfibrozil: effect on serum lipids, lipoproteins, postheparin plasma lipase activities, and glucose tolerance in primary hypertriglyceridæmia. Proc R Soc Med 1976; 69:Suppl 2: 58-63.
20. Olsson AG, Rössner S, Walldius G, Carlson LA. Effect of gemfibrozil on lipoprotein concentrations in different types of hyperlipoproteinæmia. Proc R Soc Med 1976; 69:Suppl 2:28-31.
21. Manninen V, Mälkönen M, Eisalo A, Virtamo J, Tuomilehto J, Kuusisto P. Gemfibrozil in the treatment of dyslipidaemia: a 5-year follow-up study. Acta Med Scand [Suppl] 1982; 668:82-7.
22. Glueck C. Influence of gemfibrozil on high-density lipoproteins. Am J Cardiol 1983; 52:31B-34B.
23. Kesäniemi YA, Grundy SM. Influence of gemfibrozil and clofibrate on metabolism of cholesterol and plasma triglycerides in man. JAMA 1984; 251:2241-6.
24. Turner PR, Cortese C, Wootton R, Marenah C, Miller NE, Lewis B. Plasma apolipoprotein B metabolism in familial type III dysbetalipoproteinaemia. Eur J Clin Invest 1985; 15:100-12.
25. Saku K, Gartside PS, Hynd BA, Kashyap ML. Mechanism of action of gemfibrozil on lipoprotein metabolism. J Clin Invest 1985; 75:1702-12.
26. Meinertz H. Effects of gemfibrozil on plasma lipoproteins in patients with type II hyperlipoproteinaemia and familial hypercholesterolaemia. R Soc Med Int Congr Symp Ser 1986; 87:15-21.

Vol. 317 No. 20     GEMFIBROZIL AND CORONARY HEART DISEASE — FRICK ET AL.     1245

27. Weintraub MS, Eisenberg S, Breslow JL. Different patterns of postprandial lipoprotein metabolism in normal, type IIa, type III, and type IV hyperlipoproteinemic individuals: effects of treatment with cholestyramine and gemfibrozil. J Clin Invest 1987; 79:1110-9.

28. Pasternack A, Vänttinen T, Solakivi T, Kuusi T, Korte T. Normalization of lipoprotein lipase and hepatic lipase by gemfibrozil results in correction of lipoprotein abnormalities in chronic renal failure. Clin Nephrol 1987; 27:163-8.

29. Manninen V. Clinical results with gemfibrozil and background for the Helsinki Heart Study. Am J Cardiol 1983; 52:35B-38B.

30. Mänttäri M, Elo O, Frick MH, et al. The Helsinki Heart Study: Basic design and randomization procedure. Eur Heart J 1987; 8:Suppl 1:1-29.

31. Wilhelmsen L, Tibblin G, Fodor J, Werkö L. A multifactorial primary prevention trial in Gothenburg, Sweden. In: Larsen OA, Malmborg RO, eds. Coronary heart disease and physical fitness. Copenhagen: Munksgaard, 1971:266-70.

32. Bortner RW. A short rating scale as a potential measure of pattern A behavior. J Chronic Dis 1969; 22:87-91.

33. Simpura J. Scandinavian drinking survey: construction of indices of alcohol intake. Report 46. Oslo: National Institute for Alcohol Research, 1981.

34. Mäenpää H, Pikkarainen J, Javela K, Mälkönen M, Heinonen OP, Manninen V. Minimal doses of digoxin: a new marker for compliance to medication. Eur Heart J 1987; 8:Suppl 1:31-7.

35. Mäenpää H, Manninen V, Heinonen OP. Comparison of the digoxin marker and compliance questionnaire methods in a clinical trial. Eur Heart J 1987; 8:Suppl 1:39-43.

36. Friedewald WT, Levy RI, Fredrickson DS. Estimation of the concentration of low-density lipoprotein cholesterol in plasma, without use of the preparative ultracentrifuge. Clin Chem 1972; 18:499-502.

37. Blackburn H, Keys A, Simonson E, Rautaharju P, Punsar S. The electrocardiogram in population studies: a classification system. Circulation 1960; 21:1160-75.

38. Kalbfleisch JD, Prentice RL. The statistical analysis of failure time data. New York: John Wiley, 1980.

39. Lan KKG, DeMets DL. Discrete sequential boundaries for clinical trials. Biometrika 1983; 70:659-63.

40. Lan KKG, DeMets DL, Halperin M. More flexible sequential and nonsequential designs in long-term clinical trials. Commun Stat Theory Methods 1984; 13:2339-53.

41. O'Brien PC, Fleming TR. A multiple testing procedure for clinical trials. Biometrics 1979; 35:549-56.

42. Kaplan EL, Meier P. Nonparametric estimation from incomplete observations. J Am Stat Assoc 1958; 53:457-81.

43. Cancer incidence in Finland 1982. Helsinki, Finland: Cancer Society of Finland, 1986. (Publication no. 34.)

44. Lipid Research Clinics Program. The Lipid Research Clinics Coronary Primary Prevention Trial results. I. Reduction in incidence of coronary heart disease. JAMA 1984; 251:351-64.

45. Rose G. Incubation period of coronary heart disease. Br Med J 1982; 284:1600-1.

46. Frick MH, Valle M, Harjola P-T. Progression of coronary artery disease in randomized medical and surgical patients over a 5-year angiographic followup. Am J Cardiol 1983; 52:681-5.

47. Canner PL, Berge KG, Wenger NK, et al. Fifteen year mortality in Coronary Drug Project patients: long-term benefit with niacin. J Am Coll Cardiol 1986; 8:1245-55.

48. Strategies for the prevention of coronary heart disease: a policy statement for the European Atherosclerosis Society. Eur Heart J 1987; 8:77-88.

49. Steinberg D, NIH Consensus Development Panel. Lowering blood cholesterol to prevent heart disease. JAMA 1985; 253:2080-6.

50. Åberg H, Lithell H, Selinius I, Hedstrand H. Serum triglycerides are a risk factor for myocardial infarction but not for angina pectoris: results from a 10-year follow-up of Uppsala Primary Prevention Study. Atherosclerosis 1985; 54:89-97.

51. Carlson LA, Böttiger LE. Risk factors for ischaemic heart disease in men and women: results of the 19-year follow-up of the Stockholm Prospective Study. Acta Med Scand 1985; 218:207-11.

52. Hamsten A, Wiman B, de Faire U, Blombäck M. Increased plasma levels of a rapid inhibitor of tissue plasminogen activator in young survivors of myocardial infarction. N Engl J Med 1985; 313:1557-63.

53. Leiss O, von Bergmann K, Gnasso A, Augustin J. Effect of gemfibrozil on biliary lipid metabolism in normolipemic subjects. Metabolism 1985; 34:74-82.

How to Read and Interpret the Helsinki Heart Study

As mentioned before, the Helsinki Study was a virtual clone of the Lipid Research Clinics (LRC) trial. Reading the two sequentially, one is struck by the similarities. The structures of both are about the same, and even the language is remarkably similar.

The abstract of this study describes the basic structure of the study. It is a randomized double-blind five-year trial. The results are summarized in an interesting fashion. We are given the results in terms of number per 1,000 rather than simple percentages. Because all one needs to do is move the decimal point one space to the left to get the percentage, one may wonder why this peculiar method is employed. Remember the principle that when results are presented in a confusing or unnecessarily complex way, the purpose is to mislead the reader. In this case, it is likely that the figures are given this way to make a very small difference appear larger; thus, 2.7% and 4.1% are listed as 27 and 41 per thousand, respectively.

The introductory section is brief and points out that the drug used, gemfibrozil, not only lowers total cholesterol and LDL cholesterol (LDL-C) but also raises the level of HDL cholesterol (HDL-C). There are the usual false claims that LDL-C has been shown to be a causative factor in atherosclerotic vascular disease, lowering cholesterol reduces the risk of coronary heart disease (CHD), etc. The authors also claim, "a protective effect against coronary heart disease of elevated high-density lipoprotein (HDL) has been observed in several epidemiologic and clinical studies." In fact, no such protective effect has ever been proven scientifically. A review of the references cited for this statement will reveal a few studies with pathetically weak negative correlations between HDL levels and CHD. Of course, the authors don't reference any of the papers that show no such correlation, including a British study that was the largest ever done on HDL.

The Methods section tells us that more than 23,000 men were screened. The study accepted healthy men between the ages of 40 and 55 with no history of heart disease and "Non-HDL" cholesterol levels greater than 200 mg/dl. This "Non-HDL" cholesterol is essentially equivalent to LDL-C. The subjects were randomly assigned to take either gemfibrozil or placebo. The cardiovascular end points were nonfatal myocardial infarction (NFMI), fatal myocardial infarction (MI), and cardiac death. The defining criteria for these end points were essentially the same as in the LRC trial. The statistical methods are unimportant because we will again be seeking out the pertinent data and making our own simple calculations.

In the Results section, we are told that 4,081 men were selected for the study. Only 70.1% of these men completed the five-year course. The 29.9% who dropped out were followed for end-point occurrence and are included in the final figures. Total cholesterol and LDL-C were each lowered about 8%–10%. HDL-C was raised by a little more than 10%. The end-point data are presented in Table 3, and, as in the abstract, are given as rate per thousand rather than simple percentages.

When we put the data into our own table for common sense evaluation, it looks like this:

| | Gemfibrozil (n=2051) | | Placebo (n=2030) | | Absolute RR |
|---|---|---|---|---|---|
| | No. | % | No. | % | |
| Nonfatal MI | 45 | 2.2 | 71 | 3.5 | 1.3% |
| CHD deaths | 11 | 0.5 | 13 | 0.6 | 0.1% |
| NFMIs & CHD deaths | 56 | 2.7 | 84 | 4.1 | 1.4% |
| Total Mortality | 45 | 2.2 | 42 | 2.1 | -0.1% |

There is obviously no difference in CHD deaths in the two groups, and the whole difference in the combined end points (trivial as it may be) is due to the difference in NFMIs—the softest end point. The only truly hard end point of total mortality shows *more* deaths in the treatment group, but the difference is obviously not significant. Of course, the authors give only the figures for relative risk reduction; the numbers for absolute risk reduction are never mentioned. Therefore, the authors report a 34% reduction in cardiovascular end points rather than the 1.4% in our table (1.4 is 34% of 4.1).

The authors also include a graphic representation of the results that is remarkably similar to that seen in the LRC paper. Here, the *y* axis units are given in incidence per 1000. When these are converted to percentages, they range from 0% to 5%. A completely different visual impression would be created by a graph with the *y* axis ranging from 0% to 100%, as the two lines would be nearly superimposed on one another rather than seeming to diverge.

The Discussion section is largely given over to a comparison with the LRC trial. The authors point out that the relative risk reduction of 34% in the Helsinki Study is twice as great as that seen in the LRC trial despite the fact that total cholesterol and LDL-C were both lowered considerably further in the LRC trial. They imply that the difference is due to the elevation of the HDL-C levels in the Helsinki trial. They go on to state, "In view of the growing evidence of the protective role of HDL in atherogenesis, it is logical to raise the level of this lipoprotein either by non-pharmacologic means (exercise and weight reduction) or by pharmacologic means, at least in persons with high levels of non-HDL cholesterol." The "growing evidence of the protective role of HDL" references six articles; two of these are from the early 1950s, and the only recent one reports back on the Framingham data. This is hardly a pattern of "growing evidence."

The authors are also forced to confront the fact that the greatest relative change in serum lipids with gemfibrozil treatment was a 35% reduction in triglyceride levels. Might this change account for the differences observed? Evidently not. Even though a 10% rise in HDL (4 or 5 mg/dl) warrants treatment to elevate it by any and all means, the authors' conclusion on triglycerides is that "whether the association is causal and the treatment of hypertriglyceridemia, either by dietary or pharmacologic means, is justified remains to be established."

Although the authors claim that their relative risk figures show a much greater reduction of coronary events than the LRC trial, a direct comparison of the real figures shows otherwise:

Absolute Risk Reduction

|  | LRC-CPPT | Helsinki Study |
| --- | --- | --- |
| Total Mortality | 0.1% | -0.1% |
| CHD deaths | 0.4% | 0.1% |
| NFMIs | 1.5% | 1.3% |
| Combined CHD Deaths & NFMIs | 1.7% | 1.4% |

You be the judge of the veracity of their concluding paragraph:

> In conclusion, specifically modifying the lipoprotein profile with gemfibrozil resulted in a **marked** reduction in the incidence of coronary heart disease…and furnish[ed] additional and ***conclusive*** evidence of the role of lipid modification in preventing coronary heart disease." [emphasis added]

# REFERENCES

CHAPTER TWO

(1) On the pathophysiology of atherosclerosis, see:

Ross, Russell. "The Pathogenesis of Atherosclerosis—An Update," *The New England Journal of Medicine* 314:488–500 (1986).

Stehbens, William E. "The Lipid Hypothesis and the Role of Hemodynamics in Atherogenesis," *Progress in Cardiovascular Diseases* 33:119–36 (1990).

Benditt, Earl P. "The Origin of Atherosclerosis," *Scientific American* 74:74–80 (1977).

(2) On the subject of abrupt plaque disruption leading to MI, see:

Haft, J.I., et al. "Catastrophic Progression of Coronary Artery Lesions, the Common Mechanism for Coronary Disease Progression," *Circulation* 76 Supp IV:168 (1987).

Fuster, Valentin, et al. "The Pathogenesis of Coronary Artery Disease and the Acute Coronary Syndromes" (2 parts), *The New England Journal of Medicine* 326:242–50, 310–18 (1992).

Farb, Andrew, et al. "Coronary Plaque Erosion Without Rupture into a Lipid Core—A Frequent Cause of Coronary Thrombosis in Sudden Coronary Death," *Circulation* 93:1354–63 (1996).

(3) Little, William C., et al. "Can Coronary Angiography Predict the Site of a Subsequent Myocardial Infarction in Patients with Mild-to-Moderate Coronary Artery Disease?" *Circulation* 78:9–18 (1988).

## CHAPTER THREE

(1) Kannel, W.B., et al. "Overall and Coronary Heart Disease Mortality Rates in Relation to Major Risk Factors in 325,348 Men Screened for the MR. FIT," *American Heart Journal* No 112:825 (1986).

## CHAPTER FOUR

(1) Keys, Ancel. "Atherosclerosis: A Problem in Newer Public Health," *Journal of Mt. Sinai Hospital* 20:188 (1953).

Keys, Ancel. "The Diet and the Development of Coronary Heart Disease," *Journal of Chronic Disease* 4:364 (1956).

(2) Lundberg, G.D., and Voigt, G.E. "Reliability of a Presumptive Diagnosis in Sudden Unexpected Death in Adults," *Journal of the American Medical Association* 242:2328–30 (1979).

(3) For further details on the inaccuracy of death certificates, see:

Cameron, H.M., et al. "A Prospective Study of 1152 Hospital Autopsies I: Inaccuracies in Death Certification," *Journal of Pathology* 133:273–83 (1981).

Cameron, H.M., et al. "A Prospective Study of 1152 Hospital Autopsies II: Analysis of Inaccuracies in Clinical Diagnosis and Their Significance," *Journal of Pathology* 133: 285–300 (1981).

Stehbens, W.E. "An Appraisal of the Epidemic Rise of Coronary Heart Disease and Its Decline," *The Lancet*: 606–10 (March 14, 1987).

## CHAPTER FIVE

(1) "Current Status of Blood Cholesterol Measurement in Clinical Laboratories in the United States: A Report from the Laboratory Standardization Panel of the National Cholesterol Education Program," *Clinical Chemistry* 34:193–201 (1988).

(2) Kannel, W.B., and Gordon, T. *The Framingham Diet Study: Section 24—Diet and the Regulation of Serum Cholesterol*, Dept of Health, Education, and Welfare, Washington, DC (1976).

(3) Corday, E., and Corday, S.R. "Prevention of Heart Disease by Control of Risk Factors: The Time has Come to Face the Facts," *American Journal of Cardiology* 35:330–33 (1975).

(4) Robinson, A.A. "Ischaemic Heart Disease and Vehicle Travel," *Medical Hypotheses* 23:401–7 (1987).

## CHAPTER SIX

(1) "The Coronary Drug Project Research Group: Clofibrate and Niacin in Coronary .Heart Disease," *Journal of the American Medical Association* 231:360–81 (1975).

(2) "Multiple Risk Factor Intervention Trial," *Journal of the American Medical Association* 248:1465–77 (1982).

## CHAPTER SEVEN

(1) "The Lipid Research Clinics Coronary Primary Prevention Trial Results," *Journal of the American Medical Association* 251:351–64 (1984).

(2) Zarling, E.J., et al. "Failure to Diagnose Acute Myocardial Infarction," *Journal of the American Medical Association* 250:1177–81 (1983).

(3) "The Lipid Research Clinics Program. The Coronary Primary Prevention Trial: Design and Implementation," *Journal of Chronic Diseases* 32:609 (1979).

(4) Kronmal, R.A. "Commentary on the Published Results of the Lipid Research Clinics Coronary Primary Prevention Trial," *Journal of the American Medical Association* 253:2091–93 (1985).

(5) Frick, M.H., et al, "Helsinki Heart Study: Primary Prevention Trial with Gemfibrozil in Middle-aged Men with Dyslipidemia," *The New England Journal of Medicine* 317:1237–45 (1987).

CHAPTER EIGHT

(1) Scandinavian Simvastatin Survival Study Group. "Randomised Trial of Cholesterol Lowering in 4444 Patients with Coronary Heart Disease: The Scandinavian Simvastatin Survival Study (4S)," *The Lancet* 344:1383–89 (1994).

(2) Sacks, F.M., et al. "The Effect of Pravastatin on Coronary Events after Myocardial Infarction in Patients with Average Cholesterol Levels," *The New England Journal of Medicine* 335:1001–09 (1996).

(3) The Long Term Intervention with Pravastatin in Ischaemic Disease (LIPID) Study Group. "Prevention of Cardiovascular Events and Death with Pravastatin in Patients with Coronary Heart Disease and a Broad Range of Initial Cholesterol Levels," *The New England Journal of Medicine* 339:1349–57 (1998).

(4) Shepherd, J., et al. "Prevention of Coronary Disease with Pravastatin in Men with Hypercholesterolemia," *The New England Journal of Medicine* 333:1301–07 (1995).

(5) Downs, J.R., et al. "Primary Prevention of Acute Coronary Events with Lovastatin in Men and Women with Average Cholesterol Levels. Results of AFCAPS/TexCAPS," *Journal of the American Medical Association* 279:1615–22 (1998).

(6) "Collaborative Overview of Randomised Trials of Antiplatelet Therapy: I. Prevention of Death, Myocardial Infarction, and Stroke by Prolonged Antiplatelet Therapy in Various Categories of Patients," *British Medical Journal* 308:81–106 (1994).

(7) Chan, J., et al. Water, Other Fluids, and Fatal Coronary Heart Disease," *American Journal of Epidemiology* 155(9):827–33 (2002).

# BIBLIOGRAPHY

Atrens, Dale, *The Power of Pleasure: Why Indulgence is Good for You and Other Palatable Truths.* Duffy and Snellgrove 2000.

Bennett, James T. and DiLorenzo, Thomas J., *The Food and Drink Police.* Basic Books 1994

Bennett, James T. and DiLorenzo, Thomas J., *Unhealthy Charities: Hazardous to Your Health and Wealth,* Basic Books 1994

Bennett, James T. and DiLorenzo, Thomas J., *Public Health Profiteering,* Transaction Publishers 2001.

Bennett, James T. and DiLorenzo, Thomas J., *Cancer Scam: Diversion of Federal Cancer Funds to Politics,* Transaction Publishers 1998.

Best, Joel, *Damned Lies and Statistics,* University of California Press 2001

Bethell, Tom, *The Politically Incorrect Guide to Science*, Regnery Publishing 2005

Brignell, John, *The Epidemiologists: Have They Got Scares for You*, Brignell Associates 2004

Fink, Arlene, *Conducting Research Literature Reviews*, Sage Publications 2005.

Fitzpatrick, Michael, *The Tyranny of Health*, Routledge 2001.

Gigerenzer, Gerd, *Calculated Risks: How to Know When Numbers Deceive You*, Simon & Schuster 2002.

Huff, Darrell, *How to Lie with Statistics*, W.W. Norton & Co. 1954

Kealey, Terence, *The Economic Laws of Scientific Research*, St. Martin's Press 1996

Kuhn, Thomas S., *The Structure of Scientific Revolutions*, University of Chicago Press 1962

LeFanu, James, *The Rise and Fall of Modern Medicine*, Carroll & Graf 1999

LeFanu, James, *Eat Your Heart Out: The Fallacy of the "Healthy Diet"* Macmillan London Ltd. 1987

Milloy, Steven J., *Junk Science Judo: Self-Defense Against Health Scares and Scams,* Cato Institute 2001

Milloy, Steven J. and Gough, Michael, *Silencing Science,* Cato Institute 1998

Ravnskov, Uffe, *The Cholesterol Myths: Exposing the Falacy that Saturated Fats and Cholesterol Cause Heart Disease,* New Trends Publishing 2000.

Skrabanek, Petr and McCormick, James, *Follies and Fallacies in Medicine,* Prometheus Books 1990.

Smith, Russell L., *The Cholesterol Conspiracy,* Warren H. Green, Inc. 1991.

Stehbens, William E., *The Lipid Hypothesis of Atherogenesis,* R.G. Landes Co. 1993.

# ACKNOWLEDGMENTS

As mentioned in the Foreword, I first began to question the party line on cholesterol when I noticed that the patients I was seeing during my medical school and postgraduate training did not fit the pattern described by the consensus of opinion on cholesterol. I would like to be able to say that one or more of my instructors or colleagues helped fuel my enthusiasm for seeking the truth, but alas, this was not the case. Whenever I brought up objections to the accepted theory, my arguments were usually dismissed out of hand and often in a condescending fashion.

I was, however, inspired by the writings of Dr. George V. Mann. This professor of medicine and biochemistry at Vanderbilt University was a distinguished researcher of the highest order. He had heard and read all the arguments for the Diet-Heart Theory, and he was having none of it. He said that the Diet-Heart Theory was "the greatest scientific deception of this century, perhaps any century." Dr. Mann's clear and forceful arguments encouraged me to pursue my own investigations into this peculiar theory.

My long-dormant interest in cholesterol and the Diet-Heart Theory was reawakened by the successful promotion and direct marketing to the general public of the "statin" drugs. A few years ago, I came across *The Cholesterol Myths* by Uffe Ravnskov, MD, PhD. This excellent book brought me up to date with what had been going on in the cholesterol field over the past decade or so. Dr. Ravnskov has been a tireless campaigner for the truth in this area and a great source of inspiration to cholesterol skeptics everywhere.

But for me, the truly heroic figure is William E. Stehbens, MD, DPhil, FRCPA, FRCPath. This distinguished professor in the Department of Pathology and Molecular Medicine at the Wellington School of Medicine in New Zealand has written a major textbook on the pathology of atherosclerosis and dozens of articles in the major medical and research journals. His knowledge of the subject is second to none, and his writings exhibit a clarity of thought and exposition that are unmatched. His devotion to the principles of pure science shines through in all of his works and is an inspiration.

I have never had the pleasure of meeting Dr. Stehbens, but his influence on me (and probably many others), inspiring me to adhere to the tenets of pure science, should give him great satisfaction. For that and for all of his contributions to the advancement of knowledge, I dedicate this book to him.

Ernest N. Curtis, MD

CPSIA information can be obtained at www.ICGtesting.com
Printed in the USA
LVOW03s1149091213

364510LV00005B/41/P